Manual of Clinical Procedures in Pet Birds

Manual of Clinical Procedures in Pet Birds

Cathy A. Johnson-Delaney, DVM
Exotic Animal Consulting
Edmonds, Washington, USA

Tracy Bennett, DVM, Dipl. ABVP-Avian
Bird & Exotic Clinic of Seattle
Seattle, Washington, USA

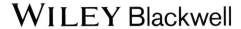

Library of Congress Cataloging-in-Publication Data Applied for:

Paperback ISBN: 9781119678137

Cover Design: Wiley
Cover Image(s): © Cathy A. Johnson-Delaney and Tracy Bennett

Set in 9.5/12.5pt STIXTwoText by Straive, Pondicherry, India

Printed in Singapore
M106048_091224

The manual is dedicated to all veterinary professionals and students who wish to be proficient in working with pet birds.

Contents

Foreword

We hope that our combined over 80 years of avian experience will be valuable to the veterinary profession. Pet avian medicine has come a long way, and many of the basics such as handling and care have evolved. When Dr. Johnson-Delaney began practice in 1980, almost all pet birds other than lovebirds, cockatiels, budgies, and canaries were wild-caught, untamed species with many health and husbandry challenges. Fortunately, pet birds now are supplied by domestic breeders, and we are not importing wild-caught birds for the pet trade. There are well-developed commercial diets, lighting and other husbandry products, and many textbooks, journals, conferences, and other continuing education available. Much of what this book aims to do is present techniques and procedures that we use in practice, honed from many years of working with pet birds. They are truly incredible patients!

Preface

The *Manual of Clinical Procedures in Pet Birds* is intended for new veterinarians and veterinary students, veterinary technology or nursing students just learning to work with birds in a clinical practice. The majority of caged pet birds are Psittacines and Passerines. If there are differences in procedure between the two, it is noted. It is organized by procedure with some general information included about the procedure as well as listing equipment needed. The techniques are described in detail as step-by-step instructions. Useful features of this manual include the rationale/ amplification sections, which may answer some of the reader's how and why questions in addition to providing information about some of the more common problems associated with the procedure. Much of this manual is written from the combined experience of the authors in clinical practice. The manual is heavily illustrated as it is often easier to see the procedure than read the script. These photographs and drawings are intended to show exactly how to physically manage the bird, equipment, and procedure. The accompanying website has some videos showing some of the procedures.

The pet bird veterinary field, including the equipment used, is continually changing and improving. Those in the veterinary profession are encouraged to seek continued education including conferences, textbooks, and journals dedicated to the medicine and surgery of pet birds. Knowledge of avian anatomy and physiology is crucial to executing all the procedures in this manual, and readers should have a basic knowledge of birds, which is beyond the scope of this textbook.

While the safety of the veterinary staff, students, and owners is a high priority for clinics and teaching facilities, the safety of the bird is tantamount. Pets can easily become stressed, injured, or even die if procedures are done incorrectly. It is up to the veterinary staff to ensure that all working with bird patients are adequately educated and trained in how to work with pet birds. It is important that restraint and handling be done correctly so that the handler is not severely bitten or scratched. Large Psittacine birds can cause major trauma to the hands of the handler or person performing the procedure. The general rule "if you don't know what you are doing, don't do it. Ask and seek help from someone who does" needs to be heeded. General information about disinfection, handling of medical waste, if different from accepted veterinary practice is noted.

We recommend that the reader uses the manual in the following ways:

- Although this textbook is designed for veterinary technicians, nurses, and students as well as graduate veterinarians, be advised that many procedures are invasive, fall under the category of "surgery," or require direction for further care. This must be done by the veterinarian. Please refer to your local veterinary medical board regulations regarding what procedures licensed technicians/nurses or laypersons (unlicensed assistants, students) are authorized to perform in your state or province.

- When the reader first learns a procedure, the entire chapter or section should be studied including the purposes, background information, complications (often listed in the rationale/ amplification sections), equipment needed, types of restraint needed, positioning, and all preparations. This background is essential for the safe and beneficial application of each procedure. If additional information is needed, the reader is referred to the list of references as well as other avian veterinary texts and articles.
- Careful attention to the rationale/amplification information can help the operator avoid common errors that can occur.
- For subsequent use, while the reader may use the technical action like a "cookbook" for doing a procedure, it is still recommended to review all the material associated with that procedure.
- Attention should be paid to all Notes (in italics) that appear throughout the manual.
- To ensure the proper positioning of needles, syringes, probes, or other equipment, the reader/ operator must attempt to duplicate the orientation of the photographs or drawings.
- It is recommended that most of these procedures be first performed on a cadaver bird, as precision and knowledge of anatomy are crucial for most. Workshops and hands-on training labs are also ways to gain practice with these procedures.

If these guidelines are followed, we are confident that the user of the manual will become proficient in a wide variety of procedures, imaging, diagnostic and therapeutic techniques.

Cathy A. Johnson-Delaney, DVM
Exotic Animal Consulting, Edmonds, WA, USA
May 2024

Tracy Bennett, DVM, DABVP-Avian Practice
Bird & Exotic Clinic of Seattle, Seattle, WA, USA
May 2024

Acknowledgments

The authors express their gratitude to the following individuals for their assistance and/or helpful comments during the preparation of this text:

Mr. Michael T. Delaney
Daniel Lejnieks, DVM, DABVP (Exotic Companion Mammals)
Grey Girl for being such a good photo subject.

About the Companion Website

This book is accompanied by a companion website:

www.wiley.com/go/johnson-delaney/manual

- Videos

1

Manual Restraint of the Avian Patient

RESTRAINT

Restraint is defined as a restriction of an animal's activity by verbal, physical, or pharmacological means so that the animal is prevented from injuring itself or others. Pharmacologic restraint is applied through sedation and/or anesthesia and is covered in Chapter 24.

Note: Restraining a bird forcibly is stressful for the bird and potentially dangerous to both the bird and the handler. Most domestically raised pet birds can be safely restrained by trained personnel with gentle handling and minimal manipulation. During all restraint, care must be taken not to restrict breathing – no pressure should be on or around the body itself, which prevents the movement of the sternum. Birds breathe essentially like a bellows system and must be able to move the body walls.

Pharmacologic agents are recommended to assist in proper restraint for (see Chapter 24)

- Procedures that are painful.
- Procedures requiring the holding of an animal in a position that may compromise respiration or where prolonged complete immobility is needed (such as for radiographs).
- With extremely frightened, aggressive, or if pain is already present.

Purposes of Restraint

1) To facilitate the physical examination, including oral and ophthalmic examination.
2) To administer medications: oral, injectable, and topical.
3) To apply bandages or splinting.
4) To perform certain procedures such as oral gavage, culturing of orifices, recording of blood pressure, electrocardiograph, and ultrasonography.
5) To prevent self-mutilation, such as placement of a collar.

Complications

- Stress.
- Overheating (hyperthermia).
- Dyspnea.
- Tissue trauma including muscle strain and feather damage.

Manual of Clinical Procedures in Pet Birds, First Edition. Cathy A. Johnson-Delaney and Tracy Bennett.
© 2025 John Wiley & Sons, Inc. Published 2025 by John Wiley & Sons, Inc.
Companion website: www.wiley.com/go/johnson-delaney/manual

Equipment Needed

- Various sizes of towels. It is recommended to avoid red-colored towels – some birds are stressed by the color.
- Various sizes of restraint straps:
- Various types and sizes of collars, including padding materials and fasteners
- Sedation/anesthesia (see Chapter 24)

Procedure

Removing the bird from a cage or carrier

Purpose

In order for a bird to be physically examined, it must be removed from the cage or carrier. It is preferable for the bird to come out on its own; however, many frightened or ill birds will not.

Technical Action

1) Most birds will come out of a cage on their own, either on a perch (stick) or to a hand. Small passerines are usually flighted, and so are usually caught within their cage or carrier.
2) Only reach into a cage to catch a bird if it will not come on its own.
3) Move slowly. Have an appropriately sized towel that is slowly introduced into the cage.
4) Allow the bird to watch and talk softly to it.
5) Depending on the size of the bird or if the bird latches onto the cage bars, you may slowly place the towel over the bird (on the side of the cage or the bottom of the cage).
6) Find the bird's head and gently use your thumb and fingers to restrain the mandible, and while moving the towel around the body, use your other hand to help secure the feet and shoulders.
7) Gently lift the bird out of the cage and reposition the towel. It is preferable to have the bird's head exposed.
8) Take care not to inhibit movement of the body wall.

Rationale/Amplification

Towel color may have associations for particular birds. You may want to talk to the owner about previous interactions with the veterinarian or other experiences if it involved particular colors, movements, and sounds.
Assoc with #4: Birds that are not used to being handled may be frightened by someone entering their cage. Dimming the lights in the exam room may help calm them. If a bird frantically starts trying to fly around the cage, back out and allow the bird to calm down. Go more slowly the next time entering the cage, and then you may need to move very swiftly to drop the towel and grasp the mandible.
Assoc with #5: if the bird goes to the bottom of the cage or into a cage corner, the towel can be slowly dropped over the bird, and then you can manually find the mandible for restraint.
If the bird is clenched to the bars and side of a cage, you may need to slowly lift the toes and get them under control with your other hand. To get the bird to let go of the cage, sometimes a few drops of sugar water dribbled on the rhinotheca so they enter the mouth will get the bird to release as it tastes the water.
Assoc with #8: Restraining the head and the feet; allowing the body free movement takes practice with many types of pet birds. Usually the shoulders of the bird are also restrained by the hand holding the mandible.

Procedure

Using a towel to manually restrain a bird

Purpose: Manually restrain a bird by grasping the mandible through the towel, cupping the shoulders with that hand. The towel can lightly wrap around the bird, preventing flapping and grabbing with the feet – the bird could potentially injure itself or the handler. Small birds can be restrained with one hand.

Technical Action

1) The bird is out of the carrier or cage.

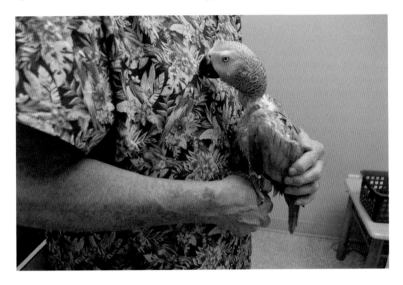

2) Approach the bird slowly, talking to it.
3) If you are right-handed, you will want to restrain the bird's mandible and head with your left; if you are left-handed, you will use your right hand.
4) With the towel in the left hand, slowly surround the bird with your hand and a towel, and then slowly with the toweled hand, secure the bird's head and mandible from behind, while bringing the rest of the towel across its body with your right hand.

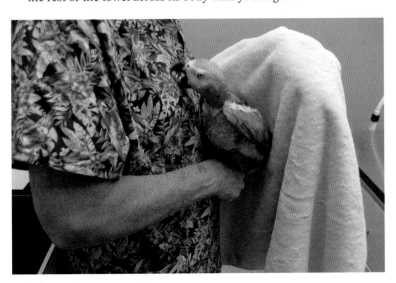

5) Once the towel is draped around, you can lift the bird off the perch or surface.
6) Secure the feet – let them grasp the towel or your jacket/scrub top. Very small birds like budgies can have their feet clasped between your fourth and fifth fingers.
7) The bird is frequently held at an angle with the feet against your body, and the head is elevated to an easy visual position for the examination.
8)

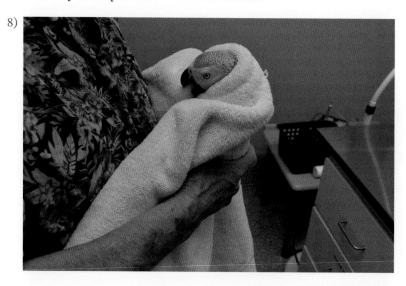

Rationale/Amplification

\# Following Dr. Brian Speer's approach as you drape the towel, often the wording is "Mr. Towel is going to greet you, and wants to hold you" . . . etc. Talking softly to the bird often calms it as they usually know their name. Do not show fear – be gentle, but not hesitant.

\# #5,6,7: Depending on the size of the bird and the type of examination or medication administration or other procedures, you can reposition the towel as needed and adjust the angle you are holding the bird. Be sure the bird does not overheat in the towel. If the bird struggles and vocalizes, you may need to consider the addition of some sedation to decrease the stress.

Procedure

Using a restraint strap

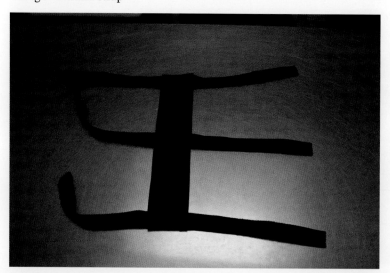

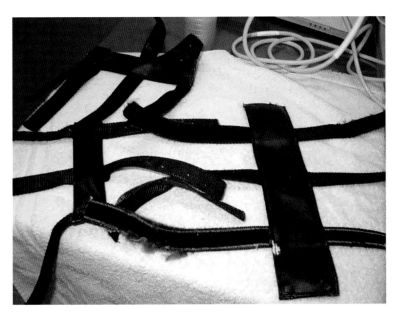

Various sizes of restraint straps

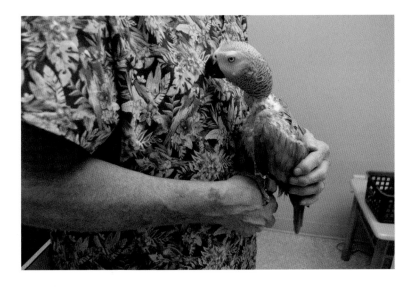

Purpose

With a bird in a towel restraint, the use of the strap allows the bird lay in the towel and strap, usually chewing on the towel, and frees the hands of the clinician to do the examination or procedures. Birds are usually calmer in this restraint than just manually in a towel, struggle less, and in the author's experience, are less likely to overheat. Restraint straps are usually unnecessary with small passerines such as canaries and finches. Larger passerines such as starlings and crows can be restrained, similarly to a psittacine.

The original design of the strap was done by Dr. Robert Shelley, Washington State University Class of 1980. Both authors worked with him. The straps are in four sizes made from stitched vinyl with three straps made of hook and latch fastening material. They can be washed and disinfected.

Technical Action

1) Lay the appropriately sized restraint strap on the exam table, with all straps laid out.

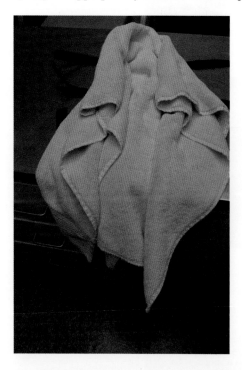

2) With the bird wrapped in the towel, lay the bird down on the restraint strap, positioning it so that the first horizontal straps will go approximately across the shoulders. Bring the two sides of the straps across the bird and secure them. It should be snug, but because of the towel, it is not constricting.

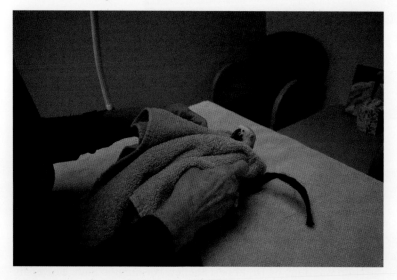

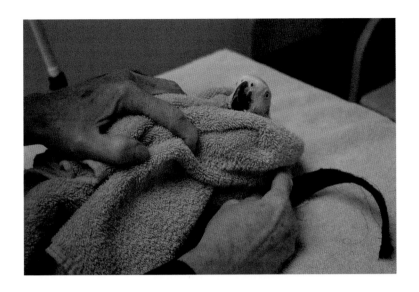

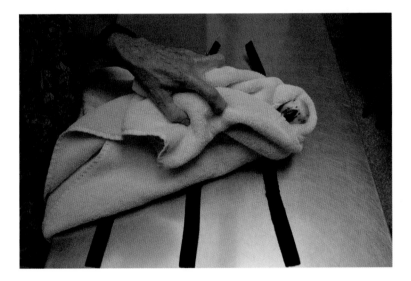

3) The middle straps are then brought across the body and secured.
4) The bottom straps are then brought across – these usually are just cranial to the bird's feet, and often the feet are within the towel.

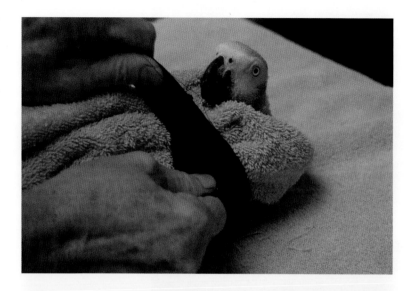

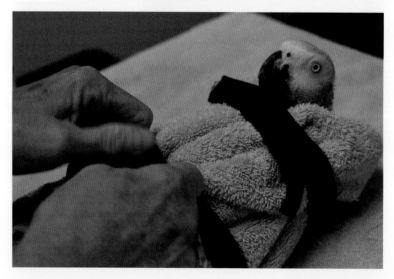

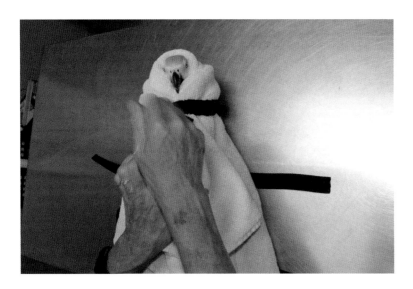

5) To examine different parts of the bird's body, the straps in the area are opened and the towel sections lifted.

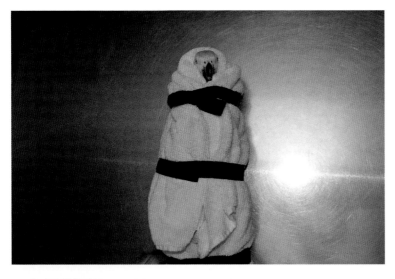

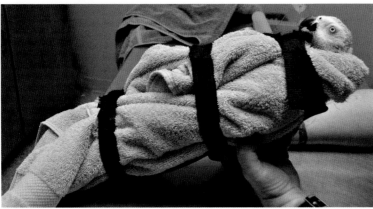

6) Some birds may wiggle down and must continue to have an assistant secure their mandible from behind the head (cradle the head in the hand).
7) Straps often need to be adjusted.
8) When finished, manually secure the bird's head and usually continue to hold the bird in the towel while each set of straps is being released. The bird then is just in manual restraint with the towel for placement back in the cage, carrier, or onto a perch.

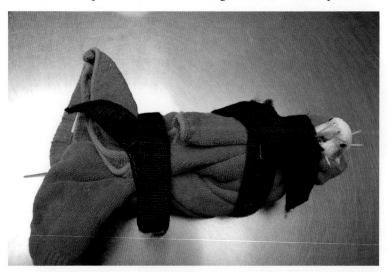

Rationale/Amplification

2: many birds are not used to being held by a human and within a towel may resist the restraint. This is considered to be stressful. When the bird is quickly wrapped in a towel and laid down on the strap, and it is secured, most birds quit resisting and instead start chewing on the towel and ignoring what is going on. The bird is less likely to be injured by trying to flap its wings, and because it is laying quietly, is less likely to overheat.

5: many procedures including full examinations, gavage, medication injections, and blood draws can be done with the bird in a restraint strap – simply by releasing the straps in the area needed for palpation, visualization, or manipulation.

8: the authors have been using these restraint straps for over 30 years and find them invaluable, especially as it allows the nurse or clinician to safely administer medications or restrain a bird by themselves, and the bird appears much less stressed than if multiple people are involved in handling and procedures/medication administration, etc.

Procedure

Placement of an avian version of restrictive collars

Purpose

For short-term restriction of a bird's access to its shoulders, breast, and possibly other parts of the body. The classic "Elizabethan" cone-type collars face down rather than up (like in mammals). Collars can be tubular (fashioned out of lightweight materials) also called "stovepipe." No matter the type of the collar, fitting one is critical, and the bird must also have supervised adjustment to it. Many birds will become extremely stressed when a collar is placed on it and should be observed closely that it can still right itself, perch, eat, and drink. One technique is to sedate a bird, place and fit the collar, wrap the bird loosely in a towel, and place in a preferably padded cage for recovery. As the bird awakens with the collar, many will attempt to remove it at first, but gradually accept it.

There are a number of commercial collars available. In general, those designed for mammals that are clear plastic with grommets and edging are heavy on a bird, and most birds can damage them quite quickly. Many collars used to be made from old radiographic film, but now various types of plastic sheeting is available. The neck must be padded and snug, so the bird cannot get its toes up under it and get caught with the foot up against the neck. At the same time, the collar cannot be so tight as to restrict the esophagus.

Tube- or stovepipe-shaped collars keep the bird's neck extended but may not prevent the bird from getting at various body areas. These can be made from a variety of materials depending on the size and strength of the bird.

Any materials used for the collar must not be toxic as the bird is likely to chew on them.

Again, most use collars only for relatively short periods of time as for post-surgery, acute trauma, or the presence of a wound. Using a collar for a chronic condition such as feather destructive disorder is usually not a permanent part of the treatment plan.

An alternative to collars are body stockings or vests, which may work better for chronic feather disorder birds. These can be obtained commercially for many of the larger bird species and can also be made from cast stockinette, cotton tube socks, or other materials.

Technical Action

1) Prepare the materials to be used for making and/or fitting a collar. This often includes a tape measure, padding material such as cotton and bandage/adhesive tape, and hook and latch type fastening tape (like Velcro).
2) Most birds are sedated and/or anesthetized for the fitting and collar placement. Measuring the bird's neck and the length of the collar and tracing/cutting the material and attaching what type of attachments and padding can take place while the bird is sedated/anesthetized.
3) Monitor the bird during sedation/anesthesia as you would at any other time. This also allows any wound dressing or other treatments.
4) Apply the collar and adjust it so that it is snug around the neck, but not constricting the esophagus. Adjust the length – for the inverted Elizabethan type; usually it should not radially stick out much further than the sternum. If the collar is made more of a cone to cover the shoulders and restrict the wing extension, the collar usually reaches about mid-sternum. The tube/stovetype – should have a normal neck extension, but not so restrictive that the bird cannot bend to eat or drink. Tube/stovepipes may rest of the thoracic inlet/crop and may inhibit filling of the crop if too long.
5) When the collar is deemed to be appropriately fitted and sized, the bird is loosely wrapped in a towel and allowed to awaken. This is done best in a warmed cage/incubator that is padded, and the bird can be observed during the whole "adjustment to the collar" phase.
6) If it is quickly apparent, the collar is not fitting correctly (like immediately the bird gets its toes up the neck and caught), or is inhibiting postures, or if the bird is getting frantic: it is best to towel wrap the bird, administer a sedative (if one is not already on-board), and calm the bird. The collar may be able to be adjusted without full anesthesia, as it will be apparent where adjustments need to be made.
7) Repeat step 5. If the collar is properly seated and fitted, and the bird is just not adjusting after 2–3 hours, a different type of collar may need to be considered or an alternative plan without a collar at all made. At this point, remove the collar and allow the bird to calm itself, supplying it with food, water, and likely hospitalization overnight, (particularly if post-surgery).
8) If the clinician is still convinced that a collar is going to be necessary when the bird leaves the hospital, the next day another attempt can be made, possibly with a different type of collar: lighter weight, smaller overall size, etc. The procedure as above would be repeated.
9) If a second type of collar fails on the second day trial, an alternative to the collar must be provided. If the second type goes fine, the owner needs to be informed about how to monitor and change positions of cage furnishings, etc. This is crucial as a bird could get caught in toys, the cage, water dish, etc.

Rationale/Amplification

6,7,8: Adjustment to the collar may take time. Some birds wake up with it on and do not appear to bother it. Others will not adjust to one, no matter the type constructed. The hazards of a collar include getting a foot caught up in it, getting the beak caught in it, chewing through one leaving sharp plastic edges, strings, dangling padding material, grommets, or other fasteners semi-attached. These can all get caught in the cage and furnishings or scratch the bird or cause further injury to the bird's body as it moves. Because of this, owners of birds with collars must be educated in how to anticipate problems and be able to closely observe the bird all day – and have it be safe at night.

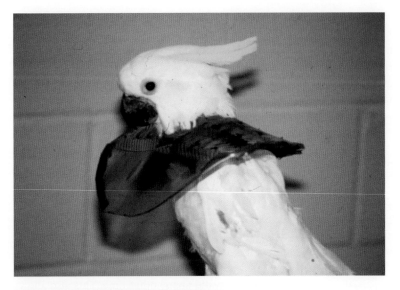

This is a soft collar made from soft vinyl

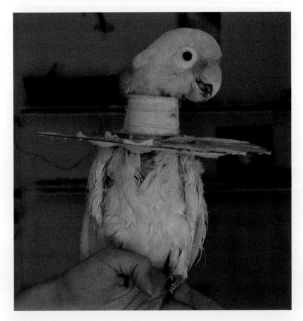

This collar designed by the owner combined the tube-type collar ("stove-pipe") with a broad E collar. The E collar part of it was removed at night.

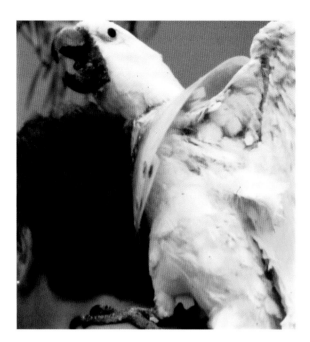

This is a commercially available collar that has snaps. Additional padding is required around the neck. For smaller birds, these may be too heavy.

Procedure

Returning the bird to its home cage or carrier

Purpose: To safely return a bird that has been restrained and is still in a towel to its home environment. Care must be taken to not entangle wings or legs/feet and also not to allow the bird to grab with its beak and potentially suffer a neck or beak injury.

Technical Action

1) Prior to replacing the bird, assess the cage as to where perches, dishes, toys, and doors are located. In some cases, some of these items may be temporarily removed (such as swinging toys and water in a water dish) especially prior to moving the cage and transport.
2) Open the largest entry of the cage as the bird is still bulky within the towel.
3) Preferably, place the bird in the towel inside the cage, on the floor of the cage, and gently unwrap the towel. Usually, you can withdraw the towel and yourself prior to the bird flying/climbing upward in the cage. If not, allow the bird to move and seek perching and then withdraw.
4) Some large birds, in large cages, that are fully awake can grasp a perch and can then be unwrapped. Some larger birds may prefer to grab the side of the cage with their beaks as well as their feet as you are releasing them.

Rationale/Amplification

1: You do not want obstacles in the cage to get the towel or your hands caught in. Swinging toys and too many perches or dishes can get in the way of the bird escaping the towel and flapping its wings. It can injure itself on any of these things in its haste to get away. A bird can fall in a water bowl and get very wet – not advisable in an already stressed bird.

3: Placing the bird on the bottom of the cage allows it to become oriented within its environment without problems of balance loss, falling off a perch, etc.

4: If the bird grabs the cage or perch with beak and/or feet, take care in unwrapping it and removing your hands. The bird needs to balance itself as you withdraw.

BIBLIOGRAPHY

Powers LV. Common procedures in psittacines. 2006. *Vet Clin Exotic Anim Pract*; 9(2): 287–302.

Turpen KK, Welle KR, Trail JL, Patel SD, Allender MC. Establishing stress behaviors in response to manual restraint in cockatiels (*Nymphicus hollandicus*). 2019. *J Avian Med Surg*; 33(1): 38–45.

2

Blood Collection

Pet birds routinely have blood drawn for hematology, serum biochemistries, serology, serum electrophoresis, heavy metal assays, endocrine panels, PCR, etc.

Most laboratories doing avian clinical work as well as in-house diagnostic equipment use small volumes of blood.

The practitioner must calculate the safe amount of blood that can be collected – more can be taken from a healthy bird than from an ill bird (Table 2.1).

JUGULAR VEIN

Equipment

- Appropriately sized needles and syringes
- Blood tubes to be used plus slides
- Cotton swabs and/or gauze pads
- Isopropyl alcohol or ethanol
- Restraint equipment such as appropriately sized towels.
- An assistant to help hold birds, particularly larger ones, depending on the proficiency of the avian clinician for holding small birds themselves.

Technical Action

1) Have the assistant/nurse hold the bird in a towel.
2) Position yourself on the bird's right side and hold the head and stretch the neck gently cranially and slightly turning the head to the left. You usually can do this with your forefinger under the bird's mandible, and your thumb is then positioned at the thoracic inlet – base of the jugular vein.
3) In this position, wet the feathers down using cotton swabs, so the vein is visualized as this apterium is located over the jugular vein. Use as little alcohol as possible to do this.
4) In this position, the vein is usually slightly raised with the digit pressure.
5) Insert the needle into the vein at its proximal position, aiming cranially. The vein is very superficial, and you will see when you enter the needle into it.
6) Withdraw the blood.
7) Place digital pressure on the puncture site as you withdraw the needle. Hold for 20–30 seconds to prevent hematoma formation. Lift your finger – if there is still some blood coming from the site, continue direct pressure for another 20–30 seconds. Lift your finger again – if no bleeding and no hematoma, then the bird can be released from restraint.

Manual of Clinical Procedures in Pet Birds, First Edition. Cathy A. Johnson-Delaney and Tracy Bennett.
© 2025 John Wiley & Sons, Inc. Published 2025 by John Wiley & Sons, Inc.
Companion website: www.wiley.com/go/johnson-delaney/manual

Table 2.1 Suggested guidelines for blood volume collection.

Species	Approximate healthy bodyweight (grams)	Approximate safe volume of blood to be drawn from an ill bird that has not hemorrhaged or lost other body fluids (like ascites) (ml)
Canary	17–20	0.1–0.2
Budgerigar	30–35	0.3–0.4
Cockatiel	100–120	1
Amazons-African Greys	400–500	5
Cockatoos – Macaws	800–1000	5–10

Source: Adapted from Chitty et al. (2018).

8) The assistant/nurse has taken the blood and placed it in the appropriate tubes and make slides, etc.
9) Release the bird from restraint.

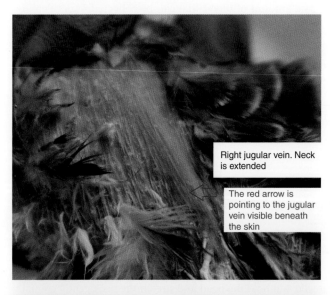

Right jugular vein. Neck is extended

The red arrow is pointing to the jugular vein visible beneath the skin

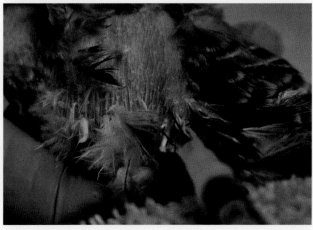

WING (BASILIC VEIN, ALSO CALLED THE BRACHIAL VEIN)

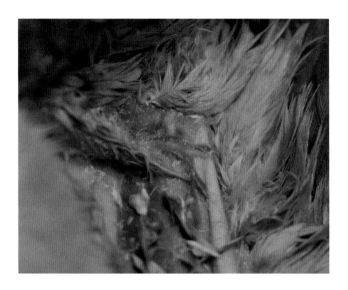

Equipment

- Appropriately sized needles and syringes
- Appropriate collection tubes and slides
- Cotton balls, swabs, or gauze squares/pads
- Isopropyl alcohol or ethanol
- Tissue glue
- Restraint towel

Procedure

1) The bird is either restrained in a towel or may be sedated and/or anesthetized.
2) The bird is placed in dorsal recumbency. If the bird becomes dyspneic or anxious, discontinue the procedure and administer oxygen. This may not be a route for this bird.
3) Stretch out one wing, holding it by the distal part or carpus. Gently lay it flat on the table surface. Wet the feathers over the distal one-third of the humerus over the elbow and over the radius/ulna so that the vein, tendons, and bone are visualized. Do not over wet as alcohol can cause hypothermia. The vein runs along the humerus. In some cases, you may need to pluck a few feathers.
4) The vein may require rising, particularly if the bird is ill or dehydrated. Press a finger on the ventral wing just distal to the shoulder joint.
5) Using the needle guard, bend the needle on the syringe to an angle of approximately 30–45 degrees.

6) With the vein exposed and raised, enter the vein with the needle passing cranially. The vein is very fragile and superficial. Very gently withdraw blood into the syringe. The vein easily collapses.

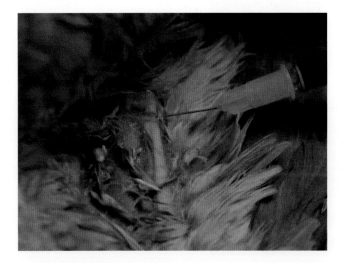

7) Place a finger at the venipuncture site as you withdraw the needle. Hold this digit pressure for 30–60 seconds.
8) Lift your finger a bit to see if there is still bleeding at the puncture site – if so, a drop of tissue glue can be used to close the skin. If no hematoma has formed, and the bleeding is stopped, the bird can be released. If there is hematoma, you may want to hold the site using digit pressure for another minute or so, or in some cases place a bandage on the site to continue mild pressure for a few hours.
9) Release the bird into a warm, darkened habitat for at least 5 minutes until it is standing. There will be a drop in blood pressure, which actually aids hemostasis. Monitor the bird for at least 15 minutes post blood draw.

LEG (MEDIAL METATARSAL ALSO CALLED THE CAUDAL TIBIAL VEIN)

This blood draw works for larger birds such as Amazons, Greys, Cockatoos, and Macaws.

Equipment

- Appropriately sized needles and syringes
- Appropriate collection tubes and slides
- Isopropyl alcohol or ethanol
- Cotton balls, swabs, and gauze sponges/pads
- Tissue glue
- Restraint towel

Procedure

The bird is restrained in a towel by an assistant/nurse. One foot is presented, while the other is held.

1) Locate the vein on the medial surface of the tarsometatarsus. The skin may need to be gently cleaned with a little alcohol on cotton or gauze to first visualize the vein.
2) To raise the vein, the assistant/nurse should grip the leg just proximal to the intertarsal joint.
3) Clean the skin again with the alcohol, and dab dry.
4) The needle should be entered into the vein distally and be directed cranially. The vein is superficial and fragile. Avoid excessive pressure when withdrawing blood.
5) Apply digit pressure on the puncture site as you withdraw the needle. Hold for 30–60 seconds.
6) Lift your finger. If there is still bleeding, dab dry and apply a drop of tissue glue. Check for hematoma formation – it may be necessary to continue some pressure on the site for a few minutes.
7) When there is no more bleeding or you are sure there is no hematoma formation, the bird can be released. It should be placed in a warm, darkened environment for 5–15 minutes while its blood pressure equalizes. Lowered blood pressure may help with hemostasis, but should only be short term.

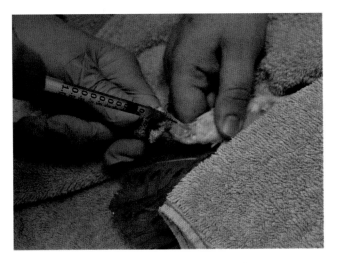

Then holding off after the draw to prevent a hematoma.

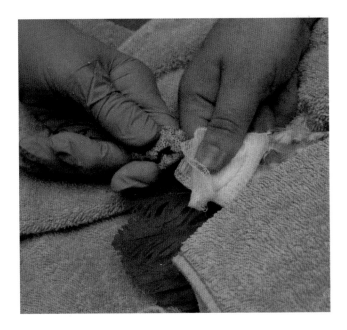

TOENAIL

While blood collected from toenails has been shown to be diagnostically fine, clipping a toenail back into the quick to achieve a good flow is considered a painful procedure.

Equipment

- Restraint equipment – towel
- Nail clippers – appropriate for the size of the nail
- Blood collection tubes, such as the kind with a collection tip, hematocrit tubes Critseal clay tray to close the tubes, and microscope slides
- Isopropyl alcohol or ethanol
- Cotton balls or gauze sponges/pads
- Hemostatic agents such as a solution or sponge
- Bandage material in case the foot/toe needs to be bandaged to maintain pressure for a few hours

Procedure

1) Restrain the bird in the towel
2) Clean a large, overgrown toenail with alcohol and cotton or gauze sponges
3) Have the assistant/nurse hold the foot out. To increase the blood pressure in the foot, hold the foot at the tarsus or even put a temporary tourniquet on.
4) Quickly clip the nail high enough to hit the quick. It will hurt!
5) Hold the foot so the blood drips freely into the collection tubes.
6) When finished, release the tourniquet of compression hold, raise the foot, and wipe the quick and apply a hemostatic agent with a piece of cotton/gauze and apply pressure for 30–60 seconds or longer.
7) The author prefers using a hemostatic sponge piece and then taping/bandaging in place.

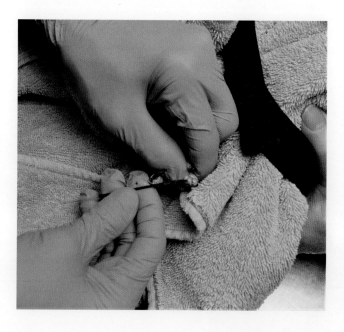

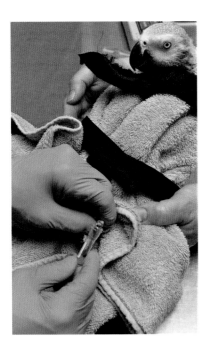

Rationale/Amplification

\# For all blood draws, apply digit pressure when withdrawing the needle. Hold for 20–30 seconds to prevent hematoma formation.

\# For ill birds and those for whom manual restraint is stressful or causes fear, sedation and/or light anesthesia may facilitate diagnostic sample collection, imaging, and therapeutics administration. This is far less stressful for the bird.

\# Despite what looks like a lot of blood from a toenail, no bird will bleed to death from a toenail.

BIBLIOGRAPHY

Bennett TD, Lejnieks DV, Koepke H, Grimson F, Szucs J, Omaits K, Lane R. Comparison of hematologic and biochemical test results in blood samples obtained by jugular venipuncture versus nail clip in Moluccan Cockatoos (*Cacatua moluccensis*). 2015. *J Avian Med Surg*; 29(4): 303–312. doi: 10.1647/2009-046R5.

Brown C. Venipuncture in psittacine birds. 2007. *Lab Animal*; 36(10): 21–22.

Chitty J, Monks D (editors) BSAVA Manual of Avian Practice: A Foundation Manual. Quedgeley, UK. BSAVA. 2018: 172–186.

Echols S. Collecting diagnostic samples in avian patients. 1999. *Vet Clin North Am Exot Anim Pract*; 2(3): 621–649. doi: 10.1016/s1094-9194(17)30113-5.

3

Injection Techniques

Injections deliver medications and fluids more reliably than those delivered orally, particularly in an ill bird that is not eating/drinking an adequate volume.

All injections will require the bird to be restrained. Intramuscular (IM) and subcutaneous (SC) injections can usually be administered easily by one person, with the basic manual restraint and with the bird awake (see Chapter 1). Intranasal administration is also usually done with the bird awake, manually restrained. For intraosseous (IO), refer to Chapter 21. Intratracheal (IT) administration is done with the bird anesthetized.

INTRAMUSCULAR (IM)

Purpose

This is the most commonly used route of injection in pet birds.

It is usually delivered in the pectoral musculature, along either side of the mid-keel region.

Alternative sites for smaller volumes can include the thigh muscles: the leg must be prevented from any movement during the injection. It is preferable to inject in the anterior thigh muscles, approximately at mid-femur.

Equipment

- Towel and restraint equipment
- Warm water on a cotton ball to move the feathers aside to visualize the muscle. Rubbing alcohol can also be used; however, it may cool the muscle which is not desireable.
- A surgical prep solution and more cotton or gauze may be needed to cleanse the skin, if for some reason there is buildup of debris, exudate, etc.
- Syringe/needle and the medication.
- Use the smallest gauge needle with a fairly short length to minimize muscle damage (usually 25–30 gauge), unless the medication is too viscous to pass through – then a slightly larger needle may be needed. The length should be sufficient to place the solution deep within the muscle body.

Manual of Clinical Procedures in Pet Birds, First Edition. Cathy A. Johnson-Delaney and Tracy Bennett.
© 2025 John Wiley & Sons, Inc. Published 2025 by John Wiley & Sons, Inc.
Companion website: www.wiley.com/go/johnson-delaney/manual

Table 3.1 Maximum fluid volume for IM injections in example species.

Species	Maximum volume (mL)
Canaries and finches	0.05
Budgerigars	0.1
Lovebirds, cockatiels, and small conures	0.2
Amazons African grey parrots	0.5
Macaws and large cockatoos	1.0
Birds heavier than 1.5 kg	1.5, deliver in several locations

Be aware of the pH of the solution to be injected. Avoid those that sting or cause pain, particularly in ill birds. Irritant drugs can cause muscle necrosis and/or atrophy (Table 3.1) (Montesinos 2018).

Volume to be Injected is based on the size of the muscle:

Procedure

1) Manually restrain the bird.
2) Part the feathers away from the featherless tract along the ventral midline of the sternum.
3) Insert the needle at a shallow angle (usually less than 30 degrees) into the muscle approximately mid to caudally along the keel).

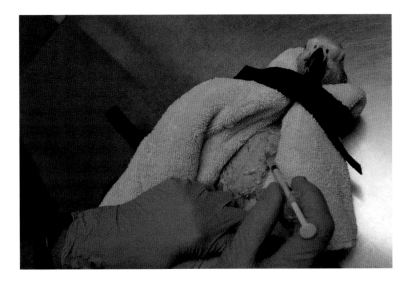

4) Prior to injecting, slightly pull back to check for blood/fluid aspiration.
5) Inject and withdraw the needle/syringe.

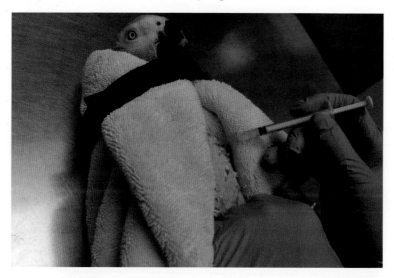

6) Slight digit pressure at the injection site may be needed if there is a small bit of bleeding.
7) Check the site for no subcutaneous hemorrhaging occurring before smoothing back the feathers and releasing the bird.

SUBCUTANEOUS (SC)

1) Useful for delivering fluids and larger volumes of medications.
2) Irritant drugs can lead to skin sloughing.
3) Volumes as large as 20 mL can be administered in a single location (depending on the bird species).
4) Sites: precrural fold (inguinal area), interscapular or axillary. Very small volumes can be placed subcutaneously in areas being infiltrated for local anesthetic procedures or, for example, under the skin in the breast area, if the feathers have already been separated for other injections (such as intramuscular).

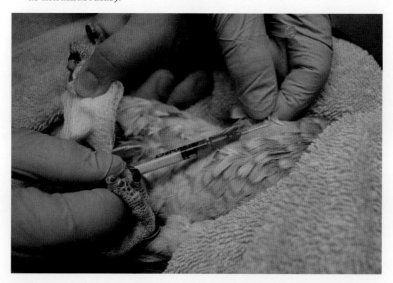

The photo above is an example of a small volume being placed under the skin over the breast muscle. This is similar to how a local anesthetic may be delivered.

Procedure

1) Restrain the bird.
2) Wet the feathers in the area of the injection to part them so that the skin is visualized.
3) Insert the needle under the skin, parallel to the skin and body wall.

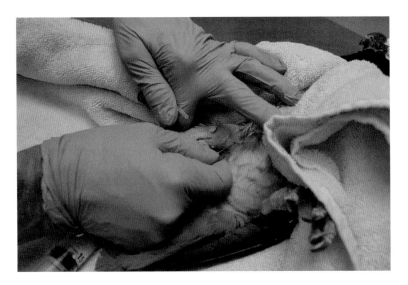

4) Inject the solution. It is easy to visualize the administration.
5) Withdraw the needle/syringe. You may need to use digit pressure at the site for a few moments as there may be some leakage (especially if given a large volume of fluid and the bird was dehydrated).

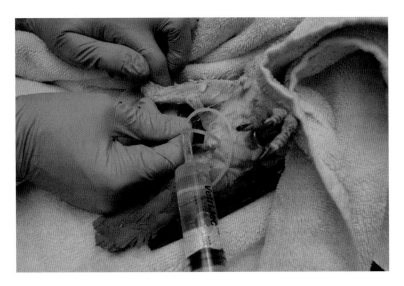

6) Check the site prior to releasing the bird from restraint.

INTRAVENOUS (IV)

1) For a single administration, a catheter may not be needed, unless it is for a slow, larger bolus.
2) See Chapter 21 for catheter placement.

Procedure

1) Single injection. The site may depend on the size of the bird, size of the vessel, and volume to be delivered.
2) Generally, the jugular, basilic, or medial metatarsal veins are used.
3) Restrain the bird.
4) Wet the feathers over the vein so that it is visualized.
5) It may be necessary to use a finger to raise the vein sufficiently for the needle to be inserted.
6) Insertion should be at an angle to enter the vein parallel to its course. Remove the finger that has raised the vein (if present) and slowly inject into the vein. You will be able to visualize the solution entering the vein.

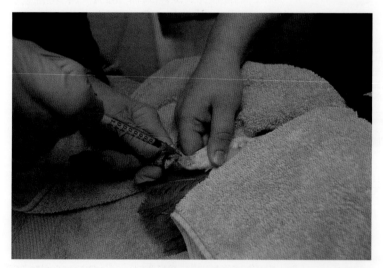

7) When finished, withdraw the needle/syringe and use digital pressure with a piece of cotton or gauze held for a few minutes to prevent hematoma formation.

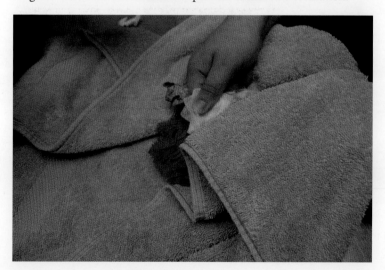

8) If there has been medication leakage outside the vein, if it is an irritant solution, then the area can be infused with sterile saline to dilute it. Be aware as it may form a hematoma, fibrose, and contract. It can also form a sterile abscess with skin sloughing. Discuss this with the owner. It may be recommended to bandage the area, and check on it daily for at least a week, treating if necessary as an open wound.

9) The following figure depicts an injection into the jugular vein.

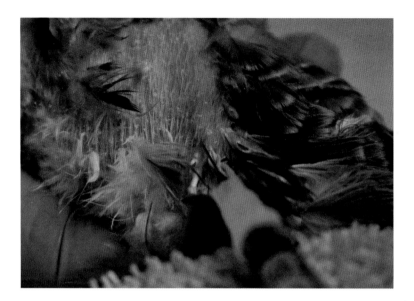

Rationale/Amplification

Do not inject into the muscle if the skin in that area is damaged or if it is an active wound or hematoma site.

It is not recommended to inject in the cranial portion of the pectoral muscle mass to prevent inadvertent injection into the pectoral vasculature.

Irritating drugs should be avoided if possible: some preparations of meloxicam, injectable enrofloxacin, doxycycline hyclate, tylosin, long-acting tetracycline preparations, etc.

Consideration of the injection sites and routes depends on the bird's condition, and how many injections and how frequently they need to be given will be part of the overall treatment plan.

Repeated injections can create hematomas and painful muscle areas.

Absorption of fluids or medications from SC sites is generally rapid – often within 15–20 minutes, although many psittacines will absorb more slowly than passerines. Check for dependent edema. Prior to any further SC, be sure that the previous dose has been absorbed.

SC fluids may be poorly absorbed if the bird is severely dehydrated and/or in hypovolemic shock.

INTRANASAL

This is done using sedatives, anesthetics, or medications delivered to treat upper respiratory problems.

The solution should not be an irritant; however, some of the sedative agents used may temporarily cause a stinging sensation or discomfort.

Ophthalmic solutions are preferred for treating rhinitis and sinusitis.

Procedure

1) Restrain the bird manually.
2) Hold the bird horizontally or slightly tilted with the head toward the floor.
3) Place the calculated volume of medication (usually under 0.05 mL per nostril) into each nostril, and hold the bird for a few moments.

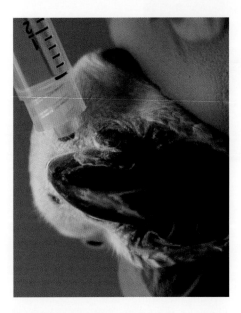

4) When returned to the upright position, the bird may flick its head and/or sneeze.
5) Wipe off any residual medication/liquid from the face, especially the feathers surrounding the nostrils and beak.

INTRATRACHEAL

This can be a route to administer medications in an intubated bird during surgery or during emergencies.

It can also be used to deliver medication directly into the lower respiratory system through the endotracheal tube.

For emergencies, a small volume of medication can be injected through the glottis in an awake bird – the bird must be restrained with the beak held open. This is rarely done.

This is also the route to do a transtracheal wash/lavage for microbiology/cytology. Prepare a sterile aspiration syringe that will attach to the endotracheal tube before the bird is anesthetized.

Procedure

1) The bird is anesthetized and intubated (Chapter 11).
2) Hold the bird upright to use gravity to allow the medication to flow into the lower trachea, syrinx, bronchi, etc.
3) Inject the volume into the endotracheal tube slowly, monitoring the respirations.
4) It may be helpful to turn the bird on its side to allow flow to enter a specific side of the respiratory system, although it is difficult to know if this is effective.
5) IT washes usually are just saline – inject slowly, allow for a few respirations, then tilt the bird with head down, and try to aspirate fluid out of the trachea.
6) If the bird shows signs of dyspnea after administration, remove anesthesia and supply oxygen. Usually it will resolve, but if dyspnea continues, you may need to insert an air sac cannula (see Chapter 19).
7) Upon recovery from anesthesia, some birds that have had IT medications or transtracheal washes will flick their heads and cough.
8) A post-procedure radiograph may help visualize if there is residual fluid.

BIBLIOGRAPHY

Montesinos A. Basic techniques. In: Chitty J, Monks D (eds). BSAVA Manual of Avian Practice: A Foundation Manual. 2018. BSAVA, Quedgeley, UK. pp 215–231.

4

Oral Administration of Medications

(see Gavage and Lavage, Chapter 12 for administration via crop tube and pharyngostomy tube)
Per os medications can include medications added to water, feed, or given directly into the mouth
Medications via the drinking water are generally not recommended in pet birds

An ill bird does not drink enough water to receive the medications.
Changes to the taste of the water may inhibit drinking, potentially furthering dehydration and illness.
Pharmacological studies have shown birds rarely achieve blood levels of medications delivered through the water.

Medications in the feed may not work in an ill bird that already is hypo- or anorectic.

- An ill bird may not eat enough to receive enough medication.
- A bird may refuse a food item that tastes differently due to the medication.
- Crushed tablets, emptied capsules, and solutions can be made and mixed with feed, using calculated dosages for body weight and estimated volume to be consumed.
- Commercially available avian feeds with tetracycline for *Chlamydia psittaci* treatment are available. The impregnated seeds may be accepted by finches and budgerigars, but the larger pelleted treated food may not be with other species, potentially leading to starvation.
- Birds placed on medicated feed must be closely monitored for consumption and body weight.

DIRECT DELIVERY OF MEDICATION INTO THE MOUTH

Equipment

- Towels for restraint
- Prefilled syringes with palatable medication
- Palatable liquids for mixing medications into include lactulose, fruit juice, or commercial compounding flavored solutions.

Procedure

Restrain the bird manually
Approach the beak from the side and place the tip of the syringe in the commissure of the beak.

Manual of Clinical Procedures in Pet Birds, First Edition. Cathy A. Johnson-Delaney and Tracy Bennett.
© 2025 John Wiley & Sons, Inc. Published 2025 by John Wiley & Sons, Inc.
Companion website: www.wiley.com/go/johnson-delaney/manual

Squirt a tiny amount of the solution into the space in the commissure. The bird will then experience the taste.

The bird may open the beak and take the liquid: squirt in the liquid slowly to give the bird a chance to swallow it.

Wait a few moments after finishing the administration to allow the bird to swallow before putting it back in its habitat.

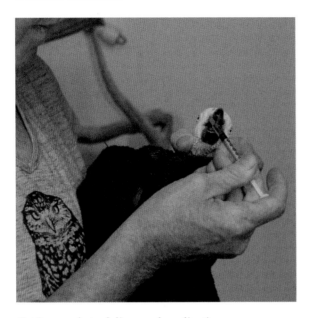

Getting ready to deliver oral medication

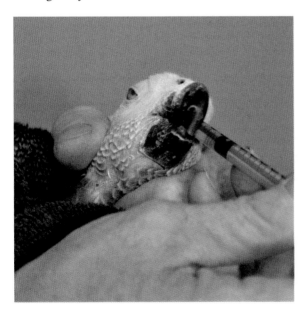

Giving the oral medication and allowing the bird to swallow. Do not squirt/force it in.

Rationale/Amplification

Oral medications are best put directly in the mouth or crop.
The medication solution should be palatable.
Birds can hold medication solution in their lower beak instead of swallowing it – when you release them, they shake their heads and the liquid sprays out.
Some parrots may not open their mouths – a soft speculum can be used; however, you likely will not do that at each medication. It is better to try and train the bird to voluntarily accept the medication.
Training can be as easy as giving the medication and vocally praising the bird
This works best on hand-tamed birds that have a bond with the owner
Classic "shaping" training can also be done but may take longer, and in the meantime, the bird must have the medication possibly multiple times a day.
Following the medication with a favored food item/treat helps positively reinforce the procedure and behavior.

BIBLIOGRAPHY

Montesinos A. Basic techniques. In: Chitty J, Monks D (eds). BSAVA Manual of Avian Practice. A Foundation Manual. 2018. BSAVA, Quedgeley, UK. pp 215–231.

5

Dermatologic Procedures

Dermatologic conditions in birds encompass the skin, including the scales of the feet, and the feathers. It also includes the uropygial (preen) gland. Bacterial, viral, and fungal local or systemic infections can affect the feathers and skin as can nutritional deficiencies. A comprehensive diet and husbandry history must be part of a dermatological assessment. Ruling out these organic causes of poor feathering or skin disease must be done prior to behavioral diagnosis of feather destructive disorder (Figure 5.1).

Procedure

Feather examination

Purpose

To examine the feather structure, detect ectoparasites and quill anomalies
From the same feather, the material from the pulp can be prepared for microbacterial culture, next-generation PCR or regular PCR testing, and cytology

Complications

- Slight discomfort as a feather including the quill base is extracted.
- If done incorrectly, it can lead toa damaged follicle that may produce an abnormal feather or no feather regrowth.

Equipment

- Surgical prep solution such as chlorhexidine 2% surgical scrub
- Isopropyl alcohol
- Microscope slides and cover slips
- Saline in a dropper bottle
- Sterile swabs – type determined by the diagnostic test to be done and laboratory preference
- Sterile hemostats
- Cotton balls and/or gauze sponges
- Laboratory tubes or containers per laboratory preference for placement of swab specimens
- Microscope
- Restraint equipment (e.g. towel and restraint strap)

Manual of Clinical Procedures in Pet Birds, First Edition. Cathy A. Johnson-Delaney and Tracy Bennett.
© 2025 John Wiley & Sons, Inc. Published 2025 by John Wiley & Sons, Inc.
Companion website: www.wiley.com/go/johnson-delaney/manual

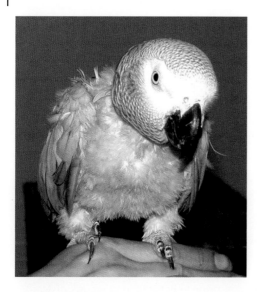

Figure 5.1 African grey parrot showing signs of feather destructive disorder. A full dermatological workup should be done to rule out other potential disease conditions.

Technical Action

1) While bird is perched, visually note the general condition of the feathers, whether the wings are clipped, evidence of feather loss, damage, and discoloration. Missing feathers and blood feathers (newly emerging) should be noted in the record.
2) Gently restrain the bird in a towel and further visually inspect the feathers, including extending the wings. Check the dorsum and ventrum, legs, neck, head, and tail.
3) A hand magnifier and light may also help examine the skin in non-feathered areas.
4) Identify a nearly grown flight feather or contour feather that contains active pulp for feather diagnostics (Figure 5.2).

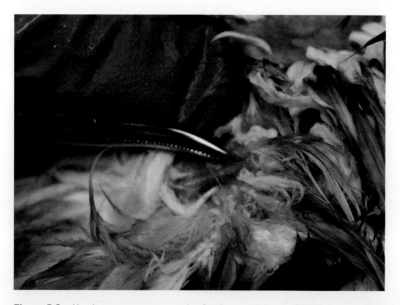

Figure 5.2 Use hemostats to grasp the feather as close to the skin as possible.

5) Gently swab the area around that feather with a surgical prep solution or isopropyl alcohol.

6) Let air-dry for a few minutes.

7) Position the hemostats parallel to the skin at the base of the feather. In one quick motion, pull the feather out. If diagnostic testing of the open follicle is wanted, swab it immediately; otherwise, place a bit of cotton or gauze and digital pressure for a few seconds to close the skin and prevent any bleeding. Figure 5.3 shows step-by-step acquisition of the growing feather.

8) If pulp contents are needed, express out for examination and diagnostic testing (see below).

9) Place the feather on a slide and microscopically examine the structure, barbs, presence of ectoparasites, etc. (you may need to section the feather for ease of mounting).

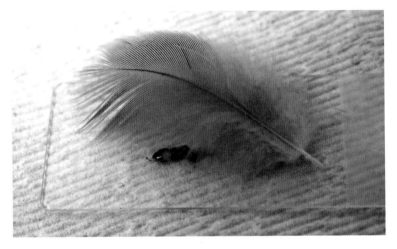

10) A drop of saline and cover slip over the feather can allow further examination.

11) If the feather structure appears to be discolored, with a material on the barbs, submit that portion of the feather for microbiology.

Rationale/Amplification

Pattern of feather loss, destruction, or discoloration can be characteristic for specific diseases, reproductive, or behavioral conditions.

+3: The entire body and feathers should be palpated, particularly for lumps in the tail area (denoting uropygial gland abnormalities) or anywhere, which might be associated with neoplasia, feather cysts, and other skin conditions. Note if there are any open lesions or ulcerations.

7: the pull is a quick "pluck" action. You want to remove the entire feather and not damage the follicle.

11: Discoloration on feathers has been linked with fungal growth on the barbs and barbules.

Procedure

Pulp cytology and microbiology

Purpose

To detect infection and/or inflammation within the pulp of a growing feather.

Complications

- Due to the small size of some newly growing feathers, the quantity of the pulp material is limited.
- Determine if the slides are to be made in-house, the material expressed onto swabs, or if the entire pulp section just put in diagnostic media per laboratory testing.

Equipment

- Surgical prep solution such as chlorhexidine 2% surgical scrub.
- Isopropyl alcohol.
- Microscope slides and cover slips.
- Sterile swabs – type determined by diagnostic testing to be done and laboratory preference.
- Sterile hemostats.
- Cotton balls and/or gauze sponges.
- Laboratory tubes or containers per laboratory preference for placement of swab specimens.
- Microscope.
- Restraint equipment (e.g. towel and restraint strap).
- Gram's stain, Wright–Giemsa stain, or other.

Technical Action

1) Restrain the bird in a towel.
2) Prepare the skin/feather base with a surgical preparation solution and let briefly air-dry.
3) Using hemostats positioned at the base of the feather, parallel to the skin, "pluck" the feather (see above Figures 5.3a–d).
4) Express the pulp material onto swabs and/or onto slides.
5) Air-dry the slides, and then fix/stain the type of staining to be done.
6) If the material was put on swabs, insert into collection media preferred by the laboratory and send for microbiologic testing.
7) If histopathology or more involved testing is needed, the entire pulp structure and part of the feather can be placed in formalin and sent to a pathologist.

Rationale/Amplification

\# 5. Gram's stains can often demonstrate bacteria and highlight types of cells. Wright's Giemsa type stains help determine the level of inflammation and types of cells present.

\# 7. Certain viral diseases may need to be confirmed via immunohistochemistry or other molecular testing, along with characteristic pathology. (such as polyomavirus and circovirus).

Skin Microbiology

Purpose

To sample skin lesions for bacterial and/or fungal organisms.

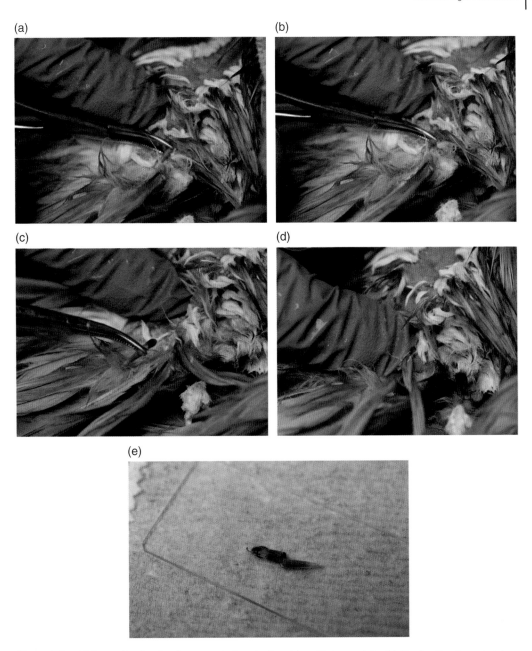

Figure 5.3 (a) A growing feather is grasped close to the skin with hemostats. (b) The feather is grasped and parallel to the direction of the feather, is quickly pulled out. (c) The feather is removed from the follicle and a finger should immediately put pressure on the open follicle. Occasionally there may be a small amount of bleeding that digital pressure for 1–2 minutes will stop. (d) Digital pressure is maintained 1–2 minutes or until any bleeding has stopped. (e) The sample feather is placed on a slide. Note small amount of blood from the base. This is material to use for diagnostic testing.

Complications

- Surface contaminants may obscure the underlying pathogen.
- Viral component will not be determined with culture and next-generation PCR sampling.

Equipment

- Restraint equipment (towel, restraint strap, etc.)
- Swabs and media appropriate for microbiological testing to be done.
- Sterile, nonbacterial static saline.
- Sterile gauze sponges.
- Antimicrobial dressing and bandage material for lesions after sampling if necessary.

Technical Action

1) Restrain the bird in the towel so that the area to be sampled is exposed.
2) Irrigate the lesion with nonbacterial static saline and clean any scabbing or debris off the surface.
3) If the wound starts to bleed a little or ooze, apply a sterile gauze sponge for just a few seconds with gentle digital pressure to dry the surface.
4) Use the sterile swabs to wipe the surface to collect the material – place in labeled tubes for sending to the laboratory.
5) For healing, comfort, irrigate with saline, dab dry with a gauze sponge, and apply antimicrobial cream (not ointment!) of choice and bandage or cover so that the bird cannot further damage the lesion.

Rationale/Amplification

3: Blood and exudate may interfere with microbial sampling, if the agent is in small numbers. Also, it is advantageous to control any bleeding. The use of hemostatic agents on an open surface is not recommended as this is painful and may inhibit healing and further damage the tissue.

Impression Smears

Purpose

To detect surface flora, including contaminants. May also yield cells to assess inflammation.

Complications

- Contaminants may obscure the underlying pathogen.

Equipment

- Restraint equipment (towel, restraint strap, etc.)
- Sterile or alcohol-cleaned and dried microscope slides.
- Cover slips.
- Stains such as Gram's, Wright–Giemsa, or others.
- Nonbacteriostatic sterile saline, sterile gauze sponges.
- Wound dressing material for covering the lesion after sampling.

Technical Action

1) Restrain the bird such that the area to be sampled is exposed.
2) If the lesion is scabbed, surface-dried, and pus present, it should be gently irrigated with the nonbacteriostatic saline and cleaned with gauze sponges to remove the debris and uncover the tissue surface to be sampled.
3) Dab excess liquid off the surface including any oozing blood.
4) Gently press a slide to the lesion. Repeat with several slides.
5) Process slides per type of the examination to be done and staining to be done.
6) Lesions may be covered with antimicrobial cream (not ointment!) and bandaging if necessary.

Rationale/Amplification

2, 3: it is usually necessary to remove dried scabbing and contaminants to expose the tissue surface to be sampled. Use only nonbacteriostatic sterile saline if microbial samples are to be taken.

FNA BIOPSIES

Purpose

To obtain fluid or cellular material for cytology or limited biopsy of a mass

Complications

- If the lesion contains an aneurysm or is a hematoma, insertion of a needle may cause hemorrhage.
- If the mass is somewhat solid or solid on palpation, the number of cells obtained may not be sufficient for diagnosis.
- If the mass is an inspissated or calcified abscess, only exudative cells may be obtained, and the sample is unlikely to be useful for microbiology.
- Inserting a needle through the skin is often painful: a local anesthetic should be injected/infiltrated through the site prior to the needle insertion.
- Forceful injection of cells and material obtained within the needle may cause damage to the sample when squirted onto a slide.

Equipment

- Restraint equipment (towel, restraint strap, etc.)
- Local anesthetic: 1 or 2% lidocaine, sterile saline diluent, insulin syringe with no dead space 29–27 gauge needle.
- Surgical preparation solution such as 2% chlorhexidine surgical scrub.
- Sterile gauze sponges.
- 25–23 ga needle mounted on a 1–3 cc syringe (size depends on the mass of the sample).
- Clean microscope slides.
- Stain: such as Wright–Giemsa. Fixative per type of staining. If sending to a lab for evaluation, follow directions for submission.

Technical Action

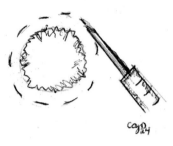

Caption: Step 1: Using nonalcohol, surgical preparation solution, cleanse the skin around and including the mass. Do a local anesthetic infusion around the mass, using an anesthetic such as lidocaine 1 or 2%.

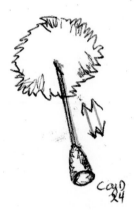

Step 2: Insert a needle into the mass. Push in and pull out multiple times, redirecting it slightly each time. This is called the "woodpecker technique."

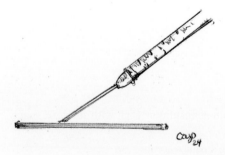

Step 3: Attach a 1-mL syringe with a small amount of air. Direct the needle against a microscope slide and depress the plunger quickly, allowing a "splatter" of material onto the slide.

1) Restrain the bird using restraint equipment such as a towel, positioning the bird so that the site to be sampled is exposed.

2) Surgically prepare the site over the lesion to be sampled using the surgical prep solution. Dab dry with a sterile gauze sponge.

3) Inject circumferentially around the lesion to anesthetize the site.

4) Dab away any slight hemorrhage.

5) There are two ways to get cells into the needle: the first way is to use just the needle and insert it into the mass multiple times, at different angles, to push cells into the needle. This is sometimes called "the woodpecker method." The second way is to use the syringe attached to the needle and use very slight suction to pull cells into the needle. There is more of a chance of damaging cells using this method, so it is not usually recommended.

6) If the sample is obtained from using the needle alone, attach a 1 cc syringe to the hub with a small amount of air and gently at an angle, push the air through the syringe to eject the material in a splatter pattern on the slide. If the syringe is attached already, you can detach it, add 0.1–0.2 cc of air, re-attach it, and eject the material onto the slide.

7) Prepare the slides per the type of staining to be used or per the laboratory instructions for submission.

Rationale/Amplification

3: Lidocaine will not damage a biopsy specimen nor the cells to be obtained. Prior to obtaining an FNA, use of ultrasound to image the mass is useful to determine if it is fluid or solid.

SKIN/FEATHER BIOPSY

Purpose

To obtain skin, feather follicle, feather base, and pulp for histopathology and definitive diagnosis

Complications

- Avian skin is thin, and if the bird is self-mutilating the area, applying sutures or glue to a skin deficit may cause additional chewing: covering/bandaging and in some cases short-term soft collar use may be necessary to protect the site.
- Feather follicles that are removed do not grow back; however, usually only 1–3 are taken.
- Wedge or excision biopsy from an active lesion may cause hemorrhage, so skin must be closed quickly and pressure/bandaging applied to stop any bleeding.

Equipment

- Restraint equipment (towel, restraint strap, etc.)
- Lidocaine 1 or 2%, sterile water to dilute: 2 to 1%, and insulin syringe with 29–27 ga needle
- Surgical scrub solution such as 2% chlorhexidine surgical scrub
- Sterile gauze sponges
- Antimicrobial cream and bandage materials
- Oxygen, appropriate size mask, and heated surface. If gas anesthesia is to be used, follow pre-surgical recommendations as per Chapter 10 in this book

- Sterile small pack containing the surgeon's preferred instruments for this: the author used a #15 scalpel blade, iris scissors, tenotomy scissors; fine tipped Olsen–Heger needle holders, and vascular atraumatic tissue forceps.
- 4, 5, or 6-0 suture. Usually nonabsorbable synthetic suture is used, fine, swaged on curved cutting needle, although in small birds, a taper point will pierce the skin for suturing.
- Tissue glue
- Sterile drape.
- Sterile surgical gloves
- Small formalin jar with cassette and other laboratory media for other testing
- Recommended: Sedation or anesthesia so that the bird is not stressed during the procedure.
- Post-operative analgesic such as an injection of an NSAID.

Technical Action

1) Restrain the bird in a towel and administer a sedative/analgesic combination of choice.
2) Return the bird to a small, toweled enclosure for at least 10 minutes until the sedative takes effect.
3) When the bird is showing signs of sedation, use the towel to remove the bird from its cage and place it appropriately so that normal respiration can occur, yet the site to be biopsied is exposed.
4) Cleanse the surgery site with surgical preparation solution as per any surgery.
5) Inject a local anesthetic to undermine and surround the surgical site.
6) Dab dry the surrounding skin with sterile gauze sponges. The surgeon should be prepped and gloved. Apply the drape.
7) Using forceps and the scalpel blade, tent the skin and nick through it. The biopsy site should include the margin of the lesion, some normal surrounding skin, and 1–3 feather follicles.
8) Using scissors, excise the skin sample.

Step 1. Cleanse and infiltrate with a local anesthetic.

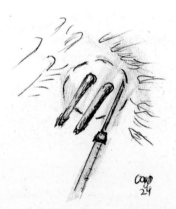

Step 2. Lift skin with a forceps and incise.

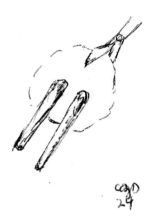

Step. 3. Suture closed.

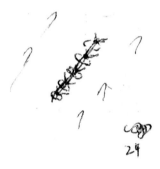

9) Place the sample in appropriate media with the vascular tissue forceps. Small pieces should be placed in cassettes.
10) Depending on the size of the biopsy, size of the bird, and the type of the lesion – either suture the wound closed or use a drop of tissue glue and press edges together.
11) Use saline and gauze to dab off any blood, apply antimicrobial cream, and bandage if necessary.
12) Place the bird in a recovery cage/incubator and monitor until fully awake. Additional analgesic/ NSAIDs may be given once the bird is standing.

Rationale/Amplification

7: Use of a skin biopsy punch in birds may damage/cut into the underlying tissue because the skin is so thin. Additionally, using radiosurgery cutting or even laser may cook/coagulate edges and in a small sample, may make interpretation more difficult. Larger samples have been sampled preferably with laser, but it is the surgeon's choice. Using a scalpel and scissors for skin biopsies causes little hemorrhage. Any visible blood vessels can be avoided.

UROPYGIAL GLAND EXAM, CYTOLOGY, AND MICROBIOLOGY

Purpose

To examine the uropygial gland for impaction, abscess, or neoplasia.

Complications

- The material within the gland normally is thick and waxy, which the bird distributes for water-proofing and grooming the feathers. The clinician needs to know which species has a uropygial gland and the normal healthy size, as well as odor.

Equipment

- Restraint equipment (towel, restraint strap, etc.)
- Surgical preparation solution such as chlorhexidine 2% surgical scrub
- Gauze sponges
- Warm water
- Swabs for appropriate microbiological sampling of the material, per laboratory
- Small towels
- Topical anesthetic cream (such as EMLA®, Astozeneca, Cambridge, UK)

Technical Action

1) Restrain the bird in a towel so that the dorsal surface of the tail head is exposed.
2) Using warm water on gauze sponges, wet the feathers on the tail head to expose the paired glands.

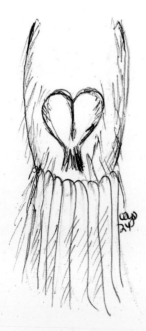

Uropygial glands paired with tufts of feathers at duct openings. Dorsal view. The head is toward the top of the picture.

3) If the glands are abnormal, they may cause pain when palpated or during expression.

4) Apply topical anesthetic cream to the surface over the glands and wait until a few minutes until the skin and glands seem to cause no discomfort. If topical cream is not enough, it may be necessary to infiltrate the area with a local anesthetic such as lidocaine.

5) Cleanse the area with the surgical prep solution before collecting any samples for microbiology. Dab the area dry.

6) Using a gauze sponge and very gentle digital pressure, express the glands pushing from craniad to caudad – a small amount of the material should easily exude from the duct(s). This can be placed directly on a swab held against the duct(s) as the material exits.

7) If no material can be expressed, a warm compress on the glands for a few minutes may loosen the material. However, if the ducts are blocked/glands impacted, they may need surgery to open them.

8) When inspection/collection is complete, dry the feathers over the glands with a gauze or small towels and return the bird to its cage.

Rationale/Amplification

\# 3: Impacted, abscessed, or neoplastic glands may be enlarged, grossly swollen, have ulcerated surfaces, and have feathers surrounding matted with an exudative material.

\# 4: Topical anesthetic cream may be all that is necessary to express a little bit of a normal glandular material. Impacted, abscessed, or neoplastic glands will require more anesthesia and likely will require additional treatments and/or surgery.

BIBLIOGRAPHY

Chitty J. Feather loss. In: Chitty J, Monks D (eds). BSAVA Manual of Avian Practice: A Foundation Manual. 2018. BSAVA, Quedgeley, UK. pp 397–408.

Paterson S. Examination of avian skin and diagnostic tests. In: Paterson S (ed). Skin Diseases of Exotic Pets. 2006. Blackwell Science Ltd, Ames, IA. pp 14–23.

6

Ophthalmic Procedures

ANATOMIC CONSIDERATIONS OF THE AVIAN EYE

Unlike mammals, birds have striated muscles in the ciliary body. They can consciously control the size of the pupil. Mydriasis is achieved using a paralytic. The cornea and globe are supported by a ring of boney ossicles. The retina is avascular, and the vitreous chamber contains the pectin, a thin, pleated, vascular, pigmented structure that provides nutrients to the retina and posterior structures. Birds with two fovea have binocular vision, such as owls and raptors. Pet bird species have a singular, round fovea. The cornea is thinner compared to that in mammals. Anterior and posterior sclerocorneal muscles control movement of the ciliary body and lens for visual accommodation.

Mydriatics:

Rocuronium bromide 1%: parrots: 0.15 mg/eye
Vecuronium bromide: African grays: 0.18–0.22 mg/kg topical; cockatoos: 0.18–0.29 mg/kg topical; Blue-fronted Amazon parrots: 0.24–0.28 mg/kg topical
Note: caution when using bilaterally. Can cause respiratory paralysis or shallow breathing, ataxia, and death. Neostigmine may counteract systemic effects.

Topical anesthetics:

In small birds, use of topical anesthetics may affect the brain; use the smallest drop possible, especially if bilateral
Oxybuprocaine 0.45%: in pigeons, with minimal side effects
Proparacaine 0.5%: most commonly used. Does not affect the phenol red thread test, may lower the Schirmer tear test, according to a study on Hispaniolan Amazon parrots

PHYSICAL EXAM

Procedure

To examine the eye using direct and indirect ophthalmoscopy

Equipment

- Finoff transilluminator
- Direct ophthalmoscope

Manual of Clinical Procedures in Pet Birds, First Edition. Cathy A. Johnson-Delaney and Tracy Bennett.
© 2025 John Wiley & Sons, Inc. Published 2025 by John Wiley & Sons, Inc.
Companion website: www.wiley.com/go/johnson-delaney/manual

- Slit lamp biomicroscope
- Mydriatic agent
- Cotton or gauze
- Avian restraint equipment such as a towel

Technical Action

1) Restrain the bird. Initially the bird is held upright, then can be laid more horizontally to apply topical drops, and then perform the exam.
2) Assess the head shape and symmetry of the eyes and note if there are any swellings around the eyes, which could indicate sinus involvement.
3) If indicated for full examination, one drop in each eye of a mydriatic agent can be applied topically.

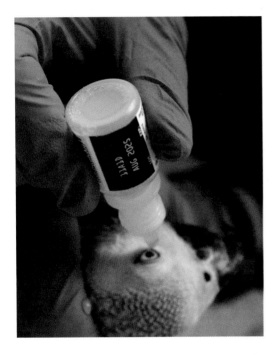

4) Use cotton or gauze under the eye to absorb excess liquid.
5) The direct ophthalmoscope can be used to visualize the eye from the cornea to the retina.

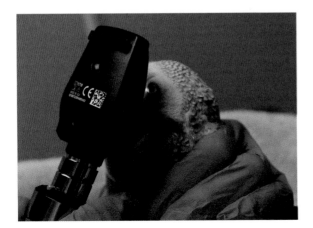

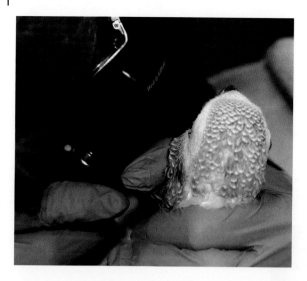

6) The slit lamp can be used to better visualize the internal structures.
7) The Finoff transilluminator can be used to visualize the cornea and anterior chamber in the absence of a slit lamp.

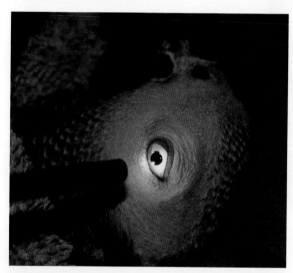

Procedure

Topical application of ophthalmic medications

Complications

- Size of the eye – many drops are larger than the corneal surface, and excess liquid needs to be removed before it drains onto the feathers.
- The bird must be held in a lateral position to put the topical on the surface of the cornea. Some birds may resist this position.
- Application of medications must be quick and the bird returned to its upright position without restraint.
- Use of ointments is contraindicated as oils can get into the feathers and cause oiling of the entire bird during grooming.

Equipment

- Avian restraint equipment (e.g. towel and restraint strap)
- Ophthalmic medicated drops
- Cotton balls or gauze

Technical Action

1) Restrain the bird in a towel
2) Hold the bird in a lateral (horizontal position), with the eye to be treated parallel to the horizon
3) Apply the topical drop to the cornea and allow the bird to blink

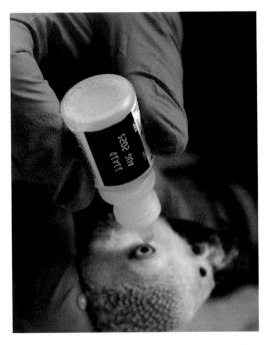

Use cotton/gauze to absorb any excess liquid before it wets the surrounding feathers

Rationale/Amplification

\# Sedation is not needed for this procedure
\# Some birds may resist this position and try to wiggle
\# Only use ophthalmic drops: do not use ointments

Procedure

Tear production assessment: 2 Methods
1) Phenol Red Thread Tear Test

Equipment

- Phenol red cotton threads (commercially available)
- Timer
- Ruler (mm measurement)
- Restraint equipment (e.g. towel)
- Cotton balls or gauze to absorb any excess tearing or dye

Complications

- There are no published values for the normal range in many species. If there is a normal bird of the same species available to test or if it is a unilateral problem, these eyes can be used as the control.

Technical Action

1) Restrain the bird in an upright position.
2) Apply the dye-impregnated thread into the lower conjunctival pocket.
3) As tears hit the cotton, it will turn red and the length of the red wicked on the thread can be measured (mm).

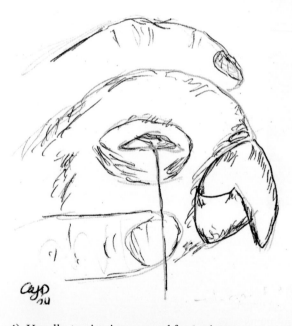

4) Usually, tearing is measured for 1 minute.
5) Remove the strip from the eye and measure the length of the strip that turned color.
6) Repeat with the other eye (especially if it appears normal – can act as control).
7) When finished, be sure to use gauze/cotton to absorb any excess dye or tearing.

Rationale/Amplification

\# The bird should be in a standing, upright position, although the test can also be done with the bird lying laterally.

\# The standardized cotton thread is impregnated with a yellow dye, which turns red upon contact with tears.

2) Schirmer Tear Test

Equipment

- Schirmer tear test strips
- Timer
- Ruler (for mm measurement)
- Restraint equipment (e.g. towel)
- Cotton balls or gauze to absorb any excess tearing or dye

Complications

- The eye must be large enough to accommodate the standardized strips. Normal values for many species are not published.

Technical Action

1) Restrain the bird (e.g. with a towel) and hold upright
2) Insert the Schirmer tear strip into the lower conjunctival pocket

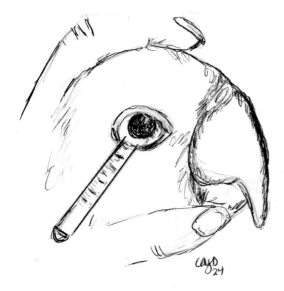

3) Leave it in contact for 1 minute
4) Remove the strip from the eye
5) Measure the length of the strip that became wetted with tears in millimeter
6) Repeat with the other eye (especially if it appears normal – can act as control)
7) When finished, be sure to use gauze/cotton to absorb any excess dye or tearing

Rationale/Amplification

\# The bird should be in a standing, upright position, although the test can also be done with the bird lying laterally.

INTRAOCULAR PRESSURE

Purpose

To measure intraocular pressure. Elevated pressure can be associated with glaucoma, hypertension, and jugular vein obstruction or compression

Complications

- Corneal irritation or erosion
- Size of the cornea
- Normal values for all species are not yet found in the literature. Use a conspecific bird or the opposite eye (if not diseased) to use as normal values for the current case.

Equipment

- Tonometer. The type to use may be a function of the size of the cornea
- 3–6 mm: Tonovet® rebound tonometer with replaceable tips

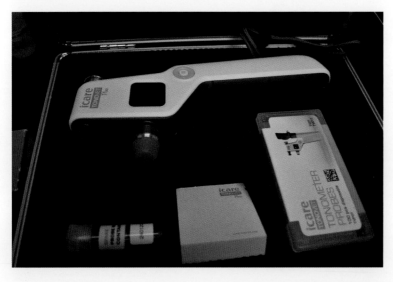

- Larger than 6 mm: Tonopen® applanation tonometer. Source: Reichert Technologies
- Restraint equipment (e.g. towel and restraint strap)
- Topical ophthalmic anesthetic
- Cotton balls or gauze

Procedure

1) Applanation technique (TonoPet®)

Technical Action

1) Apply a sterile protective tip cover to fit according to the manufacturer's instructions.
2) Restrain the bird in a towel horizontally so that the eye is parallel to the table.
3) Gently spread the eyelids, and instill one drop of topical ophthalmic anesthetic at the caudal canthi.

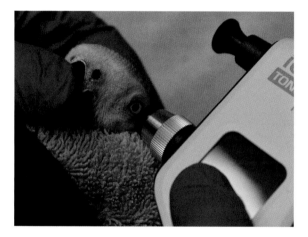

4) Let the bird blink; wait for 60 seconds.
5) Use cotton or gauze to absorb any additional liquid before it wets the feathers.
6) Use two fingers to open the eyelids fully and place the sheathed tip of the tonometer gently on the central area of the cornea. The tonometer should be perpendicular to the cornea and table.
7) The tonometer will "beep" – record the reading.
8) Lift the instrument off the cornea slightly and replace.
9) Repeat the procedure two to three times.
10) Allow the bird to be held vertically (standing position).
11) Remove the tip and wipe clean as per the manufacturer's instructions.
12) Prevent the bird from rubbing the eye.
13) Repeat steps 1–12 with the opposite eye.

Rationale/Amplification

\# #7. Usually the "beep" will happen immediately if the tonometer is perfectly perpendicular.

\# #11. The removal of the sheath, tip, and cleaning is to prevent contamination between eyes in patients.

\# #12. Use of a topical soothing ophthalmic medication may be needed if the eye appears irritated and the bird wants to rub it.

Procedure

2) Rebound technique (TonoVet®)

Technical Action

1) Insert a new rebound tip on the hand piece and activate according to the manufacturer's instructions.
2) Restrain the bird in a horizontal position, so the eye is parallel to the table.
3) Hold the rebound probe perpendicular to the cornea with your thumb on the lower button.
4) Press the button. Repeat until the audible tone changes, indicating that three readings have been accepted and averaged.
5) Repeat steps 1–4 for the opposite eye.

Rationale/Amplification

Because of very limited corneal contact, a topical ophthalmic anesthetic is not needed using this tonometer.
The probe is shooting and rebounding air on a flat plane – the reason is that it must be held perpendicular to the cornea.

CORNEAL DIAGNOSTICS

Procedure

Corneal fluorescein staining

Purpose

To determine the integrity of the cornea – traumatic lesions, infection, ulceration, etc. A damaged cornea will pick up the stain in the lesion

Complications

- Size of the cornea
- Access to ophthalmic instruments capable of assessing lesions and depth

Equipment

- Fluorescein ophthalmic dye: strips or liquid
- Sterile ophthalmic eye wash – saline
- Cotton balls or gauze to absorb any excess liquid and keep feathers dry
- Timer
- Ophthalmoscope, slit lamp, and Finoff transilluminator
- Topical ophthalmic anesthetic

Technical Action

1) Restrain the bird in a towel. Hold horizontally.
2) Put a drop of the anesthetic on the cornea, absorbing any excess liquid with a gauze or cotton to keep the feathers dry.
3) Wait 30–60 seconds.
4) Using the strip: put a drop of saline on the tip. Spread the eyelids and touch the wet tip to the cornea, usually, and the lateral canthi. If using the liquid, with a cotton/gauze positioned along the lid, put one drop of the dye on the cornea. Absorb any excess dye coming off.

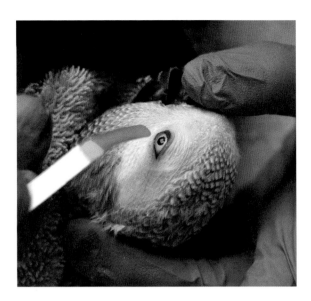

5) Let the bird blink, wait for 30 seconds, and then holding the cotton/gauze by the lower lid, irrigate the cornea well with the saline. Absorb any excess liquid to keep the feathers dry.

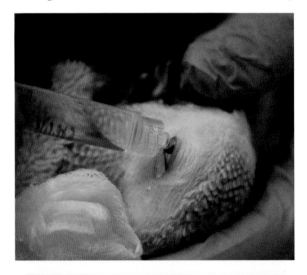

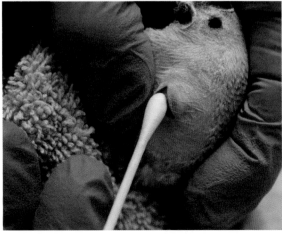

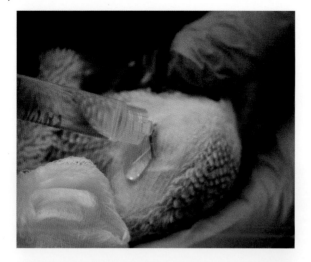

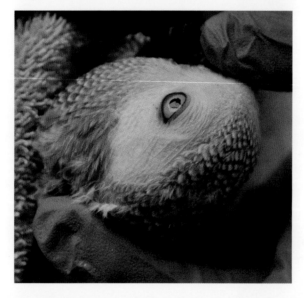

6) Darken the room, and by using the ophthalmoscope, slit lamp, and Finoff transilluminator, examine the cornea for stain uptake.

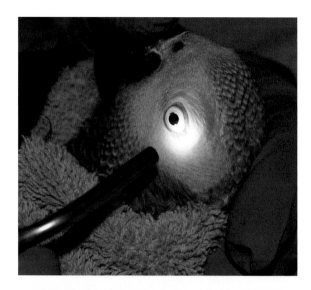

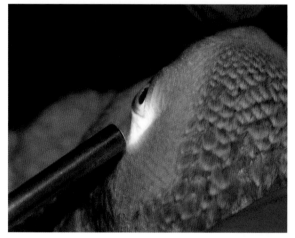

7) Reposition the bird to repeat on the opposite side if both the eyes are affected.

Rationale/Amplification

\# #2: the dye stings in either form

\# #4 and 5: prevent the feathers of the face from becoming stained and wet by use of a cotton or gauze to absorb excess dye and saline.

CORNEAL/CONJUNCTIVAL DIAGNOSTIC TESTING

Purpose

To obtain some corneal and/or conjunctival cells, tears, or mucus for diagnostic testing that can include conventional culture, next-generation PCR, regular PCR, and cytology.

Complications

- The small size of the eye in comparison to the size of some commercial swabs. Different swabs and media used will depend on the test and the laboratory.
- Because of the small corneal size, corneal scrapings for diagnostics are infrequently done and not recommended unless the bird is fully anesthetized. For common pathogen detection, this is not generally needed.

Equipment

- Restraint equipment such as a towel
- Swabs with media – depend on the testing to be done and laboratory preference
- Glass slides, coverslips, and saline for immediate cytology
- Glass slides for making smears for cytology – usually lab/pathologist prefers air-dry
- Ophthalmic artificial tears (methylcellulose)

Technical Action

1) Restrain the bird in a towel. Hold the bird upright.
2) Lift the upper eyelid.
3) Insert the swab into the lower conjunctival pouch and gently rotate the swab and move it as much as possible within the pouch.

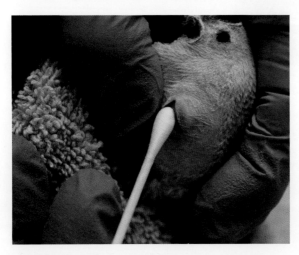

4) Remove and place into an appropriate laboratory container.
5) In larger birds, swabbing can also extend into the dorsal conjunctival pouch.
6) Repeat on the opposite side.
7) If the pouches/eyelids seem irritated after this (the bird will be having blepharospasm), topical artificial tears can be applied – one drop to each eye.

Rationale/Amplification

#3 and 4: Depending on the type of the test, there are a number of types and sizes of swabs. They usually are dry when inserted, which can cause some irritation. Avoid swabbing the main part of the cornea as that can cause discomfort and damage to the cornea.

#7: The swabbing dries the mucosa, so the artificial tears are soothing and help rehydrate the mucosa.

BIBLIOGRAPHY

Boyle JE (ed). Ophthalmic procedures. In Boyle JE (ed) *Crow and Walshaw's Manual of Clinical Procedures in Dogs, Cats, Rabbits, and Rodents*, Fourth Edition. John Wiley & Sons, Inc. 2016; pg 103–121 Ames, IA, USA.

BSAVA. In: Chitty J, Monks D (eds). *Manual of Avian Practice. A Foundation Manual*. 2018.

Hunt C. History taking and examination. In: Chitty J, Monks D (eds). Manual of Avian Practice. A Foundation Manual. BSAVA, Quedgeley, UK. 2018: pg 125–155.

Moore BA, Oria AP, Montiani-Ferreira. Ophthalmology of Psittaciformes: parrots and relatives. In: Montiani-Ferreira F, Moore BA, Ben-Shlomo G (eds). *Wild and Exotic Animal Ophthalmology Volume 1: Invertebrates, Fishes, Amphibians, Reptiles, and Birds*. 2022. Springer Nature, Switzerland, AG. pp 349–391.

Sanzhez-Migallon Guzman D, Beaufrere H, Welle KR, Heatley J, Visser M, Harms CA. Birds. In: Carpenter JW, Harms CA (eds). *Carpenter's Exotic Animal Formulary*. Sixth Edition. 2023. Elsevier, St. Louis, MO. pp 222–443.

Williams DL. The avian eye. In: Williams DL (ed). *Ophthalmology of Exotic Pets*. 2012. Wiley Blackwell, Ames, IA. pp 119–158.

Williams D. An approach to the swollen avian eye. In: Chitty J, Monks D (eds). *BSAVA Manual of Avian Practice. A Foundation Manual*. 2018. BSAVA, Quedgeley, UK. pp 317–323.

7

Sinus Flushing and Nasal Concretion Removal

Purpose

The sinuses in the bird's head are not bony, but are more like connected sacs. Nasal discharge can be serous, seropurulent, mucopurulent, hemopurulent, or purulent. There may be concurrent changes in the mucosa of the choana. The periorbital sinuses often need to be accessed directly, as communication with other sinuses may be obstructed.

Nasal concretions can form due to infections, hypovitaminosis A, and can deform the nares.

Sample collection for microbiology is recommended prior to flushing.

Procedure

Sinus aspirate for microbiology and cytology

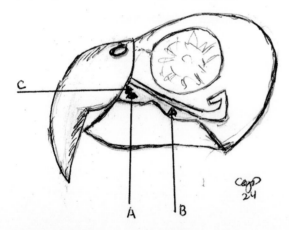

A: enter under the zygomatic arch to enter the rostral area of the sinus.
B: approach to the ventral orbital sinus
C. enter under the zygomatic arch just caudal to the beak. Direct the needle toward the ventral part of the eye.

Technical Action

1) Collection from the ventral and rostral parts of the infraorbital sinus.
2) It is preferable to heavily sedate or anesthetize the bird so that sudden movement does not lead to puncture of the eye or trauma to other vital structures.

Manual of Clinical Procedures in Pet Birds, First Edition. Cathy A. Johnson-Delaney and Tracy Bennett.
© 2025 John Wiley & Sons, Inc. Published 2025 by John Wiley & Sons, Inc.
Companion website: www.wiley.com/go/johnson-delaney/manual

3) Use a 22-to- 25-gauge needle and syringe.
4) Rostrally: insert the needle at the commissure of the beak and direct it perpendicular to the skin, just below the zygomatic bone. Insertion should be to a point between the eye and the naris.
5) Ventrally: two approaches:
   a) Insert the needle at a point ventral to the zygomatic bone, just ventral to the eye, while holding it perpendicular to the skin.
   b) Insert the needle just caudal to the commissure of the beak while directing it toward a point ventral to the eye and zygomatic arch.
6) Aspirate slowly. The material can then be submitted for microbiology and cytology testing.
7) If no fluid is aspirated, infuse a sterile fluid into the sinus through one of those access points and collect at the choanal slit.
8) Biopsies of the sinus epithelium can also be collected.

Procedure

Nasal and sinus flushing

Technical Action

1) The first sample can be collected for microbiology and cytology testing

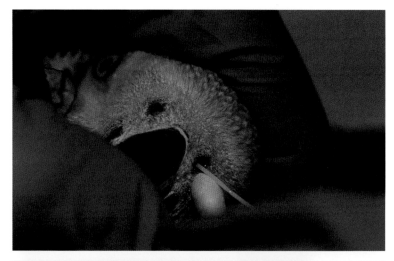

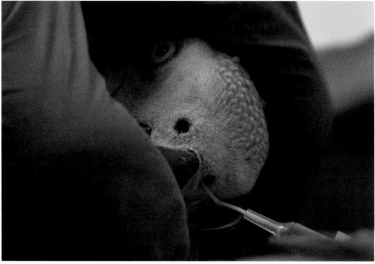

2) Because of the anatomy, only a small portion of the sinus system is actually flushed.
3) Use saline or acetylcysteine, both warmed to body temperature.
4) The bird may be held in a towel in a regular restraint position. This procedure can be done with the bird awake or mildly sedated.
5) Tip the bird forward so that the fluid flows out of the mouth.
6) Using a small catheter or the tip of the syringe covering the nostril, flush into the nares. The fluid will normally flow out the choana. Do for both sides.

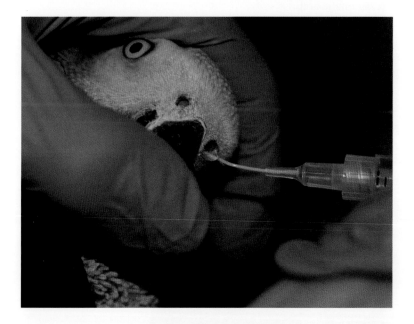

7) Allow the bird to sneeze, flick fluid, and shake its head following this procedure.
8) If the bird is fully anesthetized, it is recommended to have the bird intubated.

Procedure

Removal of nares concretions and sinus caseous plugs

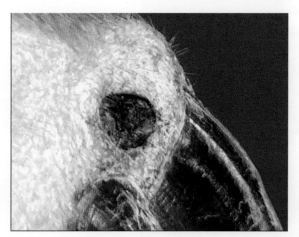

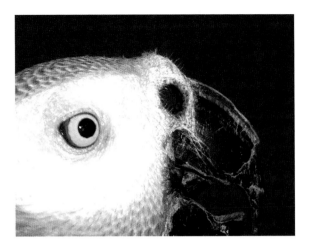

After removal. Source: Courtesy of J Hooijemeyer.

Technical Action - Nares Concretion

1) For nares concretion, the topical application first of one drop of an ophthalmic anesthetic can be used.
2) Apply several drops of sterile saline.
3) Using a small, dulled ear curette loop or dental swab, gently lift and remove the concretion.

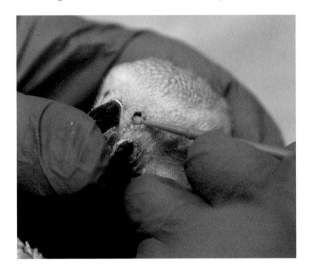

4) A micro-tipped swab for microbiology testing can be inserted into the nares and deeper into the nasal cavity.
5) The distended nares can then be gently irrigated with saline.
6) Options for direct treatment can be nasal antimicrobial drops or use of ophthalmic antimicrobials.
7) Rule out further systemic infections.
8) Discuss with the owner diet and husbandry problems that may contribute to this. Let them know that the deformation may not resolve.

Technical Action - Sinus Caseous Plugs

1) The bird should be heavily sedated or fully anesthetized. The author recommends intubation.
2) Apply a topical drop of an ophthalmic anesthetic. (in small birds, a dilute stock solution).
3) Irrigate the site with sterile saline or an ophthalmic antibiotic solution.
4) Make a small incision into the mucosa, and by using an ear scoop, ear curette, or micro-cotton tip applicators (ophthalmic sponges), gently lift the caseous material out of the sinus.
5) Irrigate fully.
6) The mucosa can usually be left open for drainage.
7) Post-operatively, the eye and periorbital tissues can be treated using ophthalmic solutions. The author likes to use a topical ophthalmic NSAID that provides site analgesia.

Rationale/Amplification

Swelling of the periorbital sinuses is consistent with sinusitis.
Nasal discharge is consistent with sinusitis, rhinitis, and upper respiratory infection.
If the nidus of the infection is not removed, the infection is likely to recur.
The entire respiratory tract should be examined as infection may not be limited to the upper respiratory system.
Diagnostic imaging procedures of the head and sinuses include radiography, CT, MRI, and with some periorbital swellings, ultrasonography.
Microbiology testing should include bacterial, fungal, and Chlamydia testing.
African gray parrots are more frequently seen with the nares concretions.

BIBLIOGRAPHY

Harrison GJ. Selected surgical procedures. In: Harrison GJ, Harrison LR (eds). *Clinical Avian Medicine and Surgery: Including Aviculture*. 1986. WB Saunders, Philadelphia, PA. pp 577–595.

Van Zeeland Y. Upper respiratory tract disease. In: Chitty J, Monks D (eds). *BSAVA Manual of Avian Practice. A Foundation Manual*. 2018. British Small Animal Veterinary Association, Quedgeley, UK. pp 299–316.

8

Grooming Procedures

Procedure

Nail Trims

Equipment

- Dremel® with low-speed control and a variety of sanding tips
- Small animal nail clippers
- Human – small or pediatric nail clippers for small birds
- Antiseptic solution (such as chlorhexidine surgical prep solution) and gauze sponges
- Hemostatic agent
- Restraint equipment or personnel

Technical Action

1) Restrain the bird (usually manually, or this may be done under sedation/anesthesia for other procedures). The foot should be held with each digit extended.
2) Cleanse the nails with a gauze sponge and antiseptic solution.
3) For small birds, manual clippers of appropriate size are fitted over the tip of the nail, and the nail is clipped.
4) Larger birds (over 150 grams, for example) can have their nails blunted using the low-speed drill such as a Dremel® with a sanding tip.
5) The trimmed nail should be checked for hemorrhage: if bleeding, apply a hemostatic agent and digital pressure until the bleeding has stopped.

Manual of Clinical Procedures in Pet Birds, First Edition. Cathy A. Johnson-Delaney and Tracy Bennett.
© 2025 John Wiley & Sons, Inc. Published 2025 by John Wiley & Sons, Inc.
Companion website: www.wiley.com/go/johnson-delaney/manual

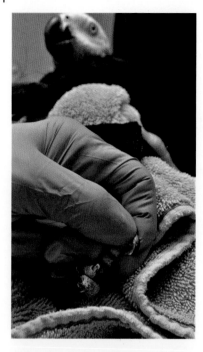

Isolate the nail and clean.

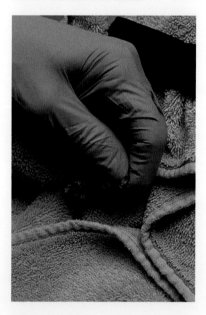

Clip just the tip.

Rational/Amplification

\# Nail trims may be necessary for therapeutic purposes beyond simple grooming.

\# A variety of perches should be available to help with natural trimming. Sandpaper perches do not work for this and should not be used as they may cause foot trauma.

Side-to-side clipping of very small nails, including that of passerines, is less likely to cause discomfort.

Bright light to visualize the central vein in nonpigmented nails lessens the chance of cutting the quick (vein and venous tissue).

Knowledge of the structure of the nail decreases the likelihood of trimming too far and hitting the quick in pigmented nails.

Nails should be cleansed prior to trimming not only to visualize the nail better but also to decrease the chance of introduction of bacteria into the quick in case it is cut.

Use of a low-speed drill with a sanding tip for larger nails is faster and less likely to cause trauma.

The popular literature promotes the use of a battery-operated electric cautery tip to cauterize the nail. While this may be effective, it may also cause pain.

Rarely a nail will need to be bandaged with a hemostatic agent to stop a nail that continues to bleed. The technique should be reviewed as it is likely the trimming extended too far into the nail.

WING TRIMS: OPTIONS

Purpose

Wing trims will not stop flight. They may slow the bird down and make it difficult to gain elevation. Some trims are done for therapeutic reasons, but most are done at the owner's request to inhibit/restrict flight. It is of most practitioners' opinion that preventing flight is not in the bird's best psychologic or physiologic interest.

Equipment

- Restraint of the bird
- Scissors – clinician's preference

Technical Action

1) There are many different types of trimming patterns.
2) The first step is to evaluate the condition of the feathers and if any blood feathers (still growing or immature) or primary flight feathers are present. These should be noted in the record and spared.
3) A pattern that has recently become popular is called the "skinny trim."
4) Pictured are different wing trims.
   A) The skinny trim: trim inside the purple line. Source: Courtesy of Dr. Todd Driggers.

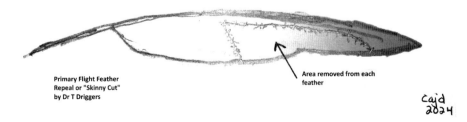

Primary Flight Feather
Repeal or "Skinny Cut"
by Dr T Driggers

Area removed from each
feather

cajd
2024

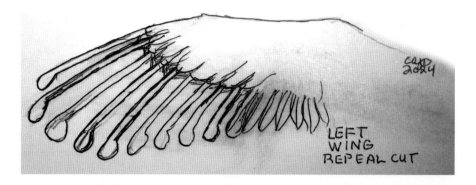

B) The tips of the primaries and many of the secondaries on one or both wings have been clipped between the dorsal and ventral covert feathers. This clip often has the cut feathers poking the bird as the wing is folded.

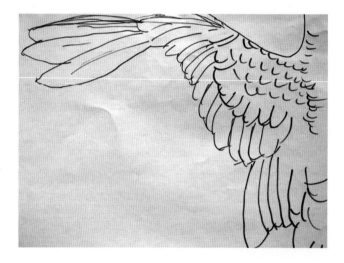

C) This is called a modified single-wing clip that retains distal primaries for some stability in heavy-bodied or younger birds so they do not crash land and injure themselves.
   a) The distal primaries however can be traumatized.
   b) Aesthetically, it may look strange to have just one wing clipped
   c) The feathers are cut between the dorsal and ventral covert feathers and may poke the bird when the wings are folded.
D) Partial removal of the tips of the primary and secondary feathers on both wings.
   a) This is the clip done by many pet stores and breeders.
   b) The feather ends poke the bird when the wings are folded.
   c) It is not aesthetically pleasing, and often this clips blood feathers as non-veterinary personnel usually do not check.

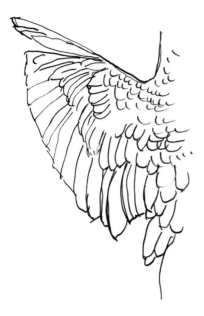

E) Clipping of all primary feathers between the dorsal and ventral covert feathers.
   a) Aesthetically, the least attractive trim.
   b) There is no protection for newly growing primary feathers, and many birds damage them in falls.

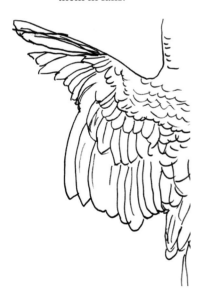

Rationale/Amplification

\# Only primary feathers should be trimmed.

\# The bird should have the ability to "brake" a descent so that it does not have to land on its keel (sternum), beak tip, head, or legs and cause injury. Landing hard can also traumatize the tail vertebrae and feathers, as well as damage feathers themselves.

\# Usually, a mature feather is left preferably one on either side of a blood feather to protect it. The owner should be instructed to bring the bird back once it is grown to revise the clip.

\# Trims should also be aesthetically pleasing so that the wings look normal when the bird has wings folded.

\# The "skinny trim" is also called the "repeal skinny trim." It is finding favor with many veterinarians if wing trimming is insisted upon.

    a) An advantage is comfort for the bird – it does not poke itself with the cut ends of feathers, and the birds anecdotally do less picking and shredding of the remaining feather.

    b) Broken blood feathers and new feathers are protected.

Dr. Bennett's preferred clip

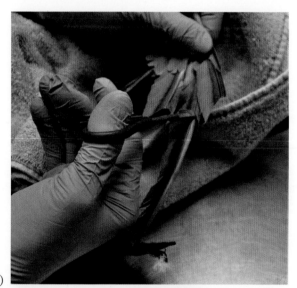

a)

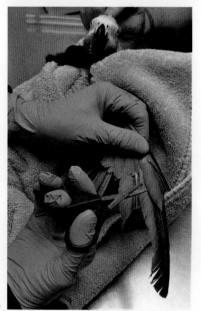

b)

c) Final result

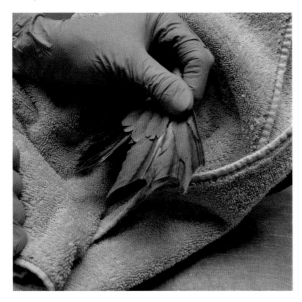

Procedure Microchipping

Microchipping provides a permanent identification system for pet birds. There are several brands, types, microchip readers, and registration companies. The chips are usually inserted through a specialized 12-ga syringe. Since the size of the needle is large, the procedure can be considered to cause some pain associated with an injection that large. There are conventions for placement of the chips, which may vary by country. In the United States, chips are usually placed in the left breast muscle. Birds with weight as less as 20 grams have been microchipped.

Sedation and/or anesthesia may be recommended to prevent the pain associated with the insertion. A topical anesthetic cream may be applied to the site first, or with cleansing of the skin, an infiltration of lidocaine can be done at the insertion site.

Technical Action

1) Restrain the bird or sedate or anesthetize. Use the best method to prevent pain and stress.
   a) A topical anesthetic cream may be applied to the site prior to site preparation.
2) Part the feathers and cleanse the skin using a surgical prep solution such as 2% chlorhexidine.
   a) A local anesthetic infiltration at the injection site can be done using lidocaine 1 or 2%.
3) Inject the microchip into the (breast muscle) chipping site. The needle is inserted in the caudal third of the left muscle mass, directed cranially so that it is expelled into the middle of the pectoral mass.

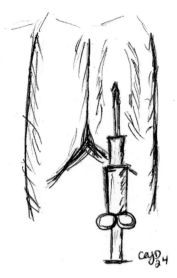

Figure 8.1 The head is toward the top of the drawing. Feathers are parted, and the skin is prepped over the exposed breast muscle.

4) The hole left by the injection can have one suture placed in it, or a drop of tissue glue, or dried and have the feathers and the skin pressed back over it. In the author's opinion, it is better to close a large open hole.
5) Recover the bird if anesthesia was used.

Rationale/Amplification

Prior to injection, scan the chip within the syringe to make sure it is functioning.
Record the number in the patient's record. Usually, the manufacturer provides some stickers or other documentation for the owners.
After the chip is placed, scan the bird to make sure the chip was fully ejected from the barrel of the syringe.
Closing the hole prevents the chip from working out and may also stop the bird from exploring a hole with its beak or foot.

Procedure Band Removal

There are many types of bands put on pet birds. The size, type, and strength depend largely on the species of birds. Many breeders will slip closed bands on baby birds, while others use open rings that are then squeezed closed. Regulatory agencies may place large stainless steel or aluminum bands bearing quarantine or other government numbers, although these are rarely seen any more in pet birds as they are no longer imported (US). Most bands have numbers that the breeder designates. Many will have the state and year on them.

Bands of any kind can cause trauma and injury to the bird – if it gets caught in the cage or furnishings, it develops infection or parasite infestation surrounding the band, or the band used was too small and has compressed/fractured the leg, etc. Most clinicians prefer to remove bands that have no regulatory function.

Equipment

- Restraint equipment, sedation and/or anesthesia; personnel to assist with leg immobilization.
- Specialized avian band cutters
- Jeweler's ring cutters
- Bolt cutters (several sizes)
- Diamond disc cutting wheel on a drill such as a Dremel® or dental handpiece.
- Hemostats (fine tipped) or jeweler's needle nose pliers
- Cotton or gauze or material to pack under the band to prevent the cutting motion from fracturing the leg.

Technical Action

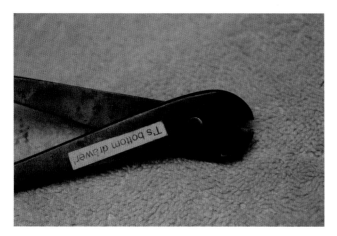

Immobilize the bird and the leg.

1) BE VERY GENTLE.
2) Packing of a soft material under the band against and around the leg should be done to prevent injury to the leg.
3) For open small bands, if there is enough space to safely grasp each side of the opening with fine tipped tools, gently open the band and slip it off

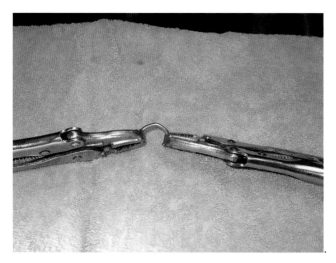

4) Another method for small bands is to make cuts in the band and then slip it off.
5) A jeweler's ring cutter can work in some medium-sized birds. It has a small lip that slips under the band, and then it can be cut.
6) Closed bands usually have to have two places cut, so the leg can be slipped out. It is critical to protect the skin and leg when doing this.

Rationale/Amplification

During the procedure, protect the leg and the leg skin from not only the cutting tools but also the sharp ends of a band.
If the skin is lacerated and begins to bleed, use a hemostatic agent and direct pressure to stop any bleeding. Antibiotic cream and a short-term bandage may be needed.
Practicing removal of bands on cadaver birds is recommended so you become familiar with the amount of pressure needed to cut and remove the bands without injuring the bird.

Procedure Beak Trimming

Beak trims are usually needed as a medical/surgical treatment as with the healthy bird, and with the appropriate diet and husbandry, beak growth should not require routine trimming. A medical/surgical reason to do so is beyond the scope of this techniques text.

Birds that require regular trims due to deformity and previous injuries causing incorrect alignment can usually be done with the bird awake and restrained manually (towel and handler). Birds that have to have this done frequently become very used to the procedure.

To properly do the lower beak (rhamphotheca), you do need to have the mouth open. This can be done using a soft speculum (such as a syringe case) or if an assistant can have a gauze bandage material around the upper beak (rhinotheca) and gently elevate so that the mouth is open. Metal speculums may cause damage to the outer walls of the beak and are generally not needed.

Equipment

- Dremel®/drill with low/high speed and multiple types of sanding and abrading tips. The use of a cutting disc may be needed, but there can be a risk of cutting into the quick of the beak and causing hemorrhage.
- Restraint equipment or sedation/anesthesia.
- Hemostatic agent.

Technical Action

1) Restrain the bird.
2) Have assistance in opening the bird's mouth to shape the rhamphotheca.
3) Remove excess beak material and shape the beak to normal conformation or as close as possible.

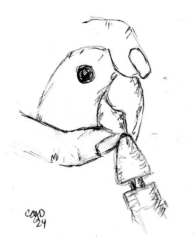

Step 1 – larger sanding tip and coarser grit.

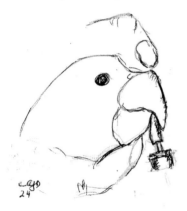

Step 2 – finishing with finer grit and smaller cone to approximate a normal beak conformation.

4) Be aware of any heat generated by the sanding or cutting tips on the drill and stop before the beak is heated.
5) Wipe away excess dust generated by the beak shaping.
6) If bleeding was encountered, use the hemostatic agent and direct pressure until it has stopped.
7) Determine that the beak shape is correct by manually closing the beak and observing.
8) Determine that if the beak did bleed, that it has stopped, and that there is no lingering pain.

Rationale/Amplification

\# The beak is a sensitive organ, and to cut into it and draw blood is likely painful.

\# Nail clippers or other cutting devices that cause torque to cut are not recommended as they can damage the germinal tissue, in addition to likely cutting into the quick or causing pain.

\# Blunting of the tip is often requested by owners who think that will make bites less painful – the bird will quickly re-sharpen the beak.

BIBLIOGRAPHY

Greenacre CB, Gerhardt L. Psittacine and passerine birds. In: Ballard B, Cheek R (eds). *Exotic Animal Medicine for the Veterinary Technician*. Third Edition. 2017. Wiley Blackwell, Ames, IA. pp 100–142.

Montisinos A. Basic techniques. In: Chitty J, Monks D (eds). *BSAVA Manual of Avian Practice. A Foundation Manual*. 2018. British Small Animal Veterinary Association, Quedgeley, UK. pp 215–241.

9

Cloacal Procedures

The cloaca of the bird is a complex organ. The colon, ureters, and reproductive tracts enter into it. In the immature bird, the cloaca also contains the lymphoid tissue – the Bursa of Fabricius. It is a bell-shaped dilation of the end of the rectum consisting of the coprodeum, urodeum, and proctodeum. In male birds, it lies midline, but in mature female birds, the enlarged left oviduct pushes it to the right.

The coprodeum is the cranial portion where the rectum empties – essentially an extension of the colon. It can be a site of water resorption. The coprourodeal fold separates it from the urodeum. When the rectum contains feces, it can bulge out the vent to defecate, without mixing with urine or urates. The fold closes during egg-laying to prevent feces being expelled with an egg.

The urodeum is separated from the other compartments by circular mucosal folds. Both the ureters and genital ducts empty into its dorsal wall.

The proctodeum is a short compartment separated from the urodeum by the uroproctodeal fold. It empties into the vent. The Bursa of Fabricius is located in its dorsal wall.

The vent itself is the external opening of the cloaca and is controlled by an external anal sphincter. In psittacines, it is a circular opening but can appear transverse in other species.

Cloacal diagnostic procedures: microbiology, cytology, flushing for cleansing, and preparation for endoscopy.

Procedure Collection of Diagnostic Material

Collection of the diagnostic material for parasitology, microbiology, and/or cytology

Equipment

- Sterile cotton swabs
- Culture tubes
- Fecal collection containers
- Sterile saline and
- Slides.

Technical Action

1) With the bird is restrained in a towel, and in dorsal recumbency, the vent can be accessed with swabs or soft catheters for diagnostic collection.

Manual of Clinical Procedures in Pet Birds, First Edition. Cathy A. Johnson-Delaney and Tracy Bennett.
© 2025 John Wiley & Sons, Inc. Published 2025 by John Wiley & Sons, Inc.
Companion website: www.wiley.com/go/johnson-delaney/manual

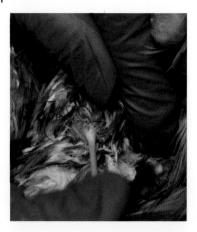

2) If resistance is met at the sphincter, application of a drop of lidocaine 2% or a small amount of lidocaine dental gel may help it relax.

3) If blood is found on any swab or in the draining/collected irrigation solution, consider inserting a small catheter and instilling a small amount of antibiotic cream. Do not use oil-based ointments on birds.

4) Check the next urination/defecation for signs of hemorrhage. If present, further treatment may be warranted.

Rationale/Amplification

\# Be gentle when inserting swabs or aspiration catheters into the cloaca as it is a functional organ.

\# Dilation for visualization can be done with the bird sedated/anesthetized, in dorsal recumbency. The author uses an ophthalmic eyelid retractor to gently open the sphincter. A drop of lidocaine gel on the sphincter can relax it.

\# A small amount of blood on the feces/urine/urates immediately after swabbing may occur, but it should not continue. Check the vent, vent feathers, and watch subsequent defecation/urination. Continued hemorrhage can be associated with cloacitis or hemorrhage in any of the systems emptying into the cloaca. Further exploration may be necessary.

Procedure Cloacal Endoscopic Examination

Preparation of the cloaca for endoscopic examination

Purpose

To examination inside the cloaca for irritation, inflammation, hemorrhage, infection, or neoplasia.

Equipment

- Sterile saline with a drip set
- Catheter such as shortened red rubber French at least 12-14 ga or other blunt catheter that can be attached to drip set
- Sedatives, anesthesia: as for surgery
- Endoscopic equipment
- Towels
- Warming system for the fluids
- Gauze sponges

Technical Action

1) Warm a 500–1000 mL-bag of sterile saline. Attach a drip set.
2) Attach a small catheter (such as a shortened red rubber French, usually at least 12–14 ga, with the edges blunted or a Slippery Sam urinary catheter or the plastic portion of an IV catheter) to the end of the drip set.
3) Sedate and/or anesthetize the bird as endoscopy may take some time.
4) Have towels or an absorbent material over the birds' tail to prevent soaking of the feathers and bird (and the endoscopist!)
5) Apply a topical anesthetic to the vent.
6) Gently retract/spread the vent.
7) Irrigate with the warmed fluids, regulating the flow with the drip set. Once the vent is cleared for fecal/urinary material and is filled with fluid, the retractor may be removed, while a low flow of irrigation continues.

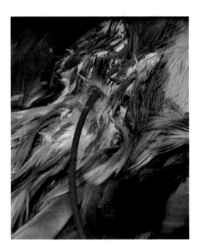

8) The endoscope can be inserted into the fluid-filled cloaca.
9) Dry the vent and the feathers with towels.
10) Recover the bird.

Rationale/Amplification

Endoscopic examination of the cloaca is essential in cases of papillomas, hemorrhage, chronic cloacitis, diarrhea, and reproductive tract disorders. You can also observe passage of urine, urates, and functioning of the cloaca.

BIBLIOGRAPHY

Bowles HL, Odberg E, Harrison GJ, Kottwitz JJ. Surgical resolution of soft tissue disorders. In: Harrison GJ, Lightfoot TL (eds). *Clinical Avian Medicine Volume II*. 2006. Spix Publishing, Inc., Palm Beach, FL. Pp 775–829.

Hunt C. History taking and examination. In: Chitty J, Monks D (eds). *BSAVA Manual of Avian Practice. A Foundation Manual*. 2018. British Small Animal Veterinary Association, Quedgeley, UK. pp 125–155.

10

Surgery Preparations

Most small animal clinics have a surgery suite that is readily adaptable for avian surgeries. The key for success is having trained staff who understand the avian patient's anatomy and physiology and have experience with anesthesia and surgical patient monitoring.

Equipment for monitoring needs to be capable of handling the higher heart and respiration rates of birds, along with the smaller size and weight. Great attention is paid to thermal regulation, as a bird loses a lot of body heat through respiration: inhalant anesthetic gases can dangerously lower a bird's body temperature over the course of the anesthesia.

Before a bird is admitted for surgery, a discussion with the owner is critical. The veterinarian must discuss the anesthetic risk and ways with which the team will minimize risk. A discussion of options along with detailing what the anesthesia and surgery will entail must be approved by the owner. An anesthesia and surgery consent forms should be detailed and signed by both the owner and the veterinarian.

Procedure

Preparation of the surgical suite and avian patient

Purpose

To minimize patient risk of anesthesia and surgery and maximize success of recovery.

Complications

- Untrained, inexperienced personnel
- Lack of warming systems suitable for birds
- Lack of monitoring equipment that is too large or not sensitive enough to handle the higher heart and respiration rates.
- Lack of a safe, warming recovery cage/incubator
- Lack of an avian-equipped crash or emergency cart or kit (Chapter 20)
- Lack of avian-sized masks and endotracheal tubes

Equipment

- A surgery table that can be elevated for ergonomic surgery. A wedge pad to allow elevation of the head (optional – can do this with folded towels)
- Operating microscope – extremely useful for microsurgery
- Head loupes or optical magnification for the surgeon and assistant

Manual of Clinical Procedures in Pet Birds, First Edition. Cathy A. Johnson-Delaney and Tracy Bennett.
© 2025 John Wiley & Sons, Inc. Published 2025 by John Wiley & Sons, Inc.
Companion website: www.wiley.com/go/johnson-delaney/manual

- Microsurgery, avian-sized surgical instruments, sterilized.
- Syringe pump
- Vitals monitoring equipment: ECG, blood pressure (need neonatal, small cuffs), pulse oximetry, side-stream capnographic sensor, thermometer (electronic), stethoscope (electronic for amplification), and audio Doppler system.
- Radiosurgery unit and/or surgical laser system
- Anesthesia machine with a vaporizer for inhalant anesthesia and oxygen
- Ventilator – one that can do exotics or neonatal cats/dogs.
- Masks, endotracheal tubes, without cuffs of appropriate sizes; plus supplies to be able to tie in/ secure the mask/endotracheal tube.
- Emergency – crash cart or kit
- Tape, gauze strips, and gauze sponges
- Catheters, fluid delivery system, and fluids. A warming system for fluids is recommended.
- Surgical scrub solution such as 2% chlorhexidine surgical scrub
- Surgical instrument packs, sterile clear adhesive drape, sterile gauze, and any specialty tools required.
- Endoscopic system
- Formulary
- Calculator
- Checklists and spreadsheets for vitals recording.
- Needles and syringes of various sizes
- Warmed fluids and saline
- Sterile surgical gloves, gowns, shoe covers, hair covers, and masks as per any aseptic surgery
- The surgical suite itself may be kept slightly warmer than other rooms for bird work.
- Recovery cage, incubator, or critical care-type caging that can be kept warm and oxygen can be supplied.

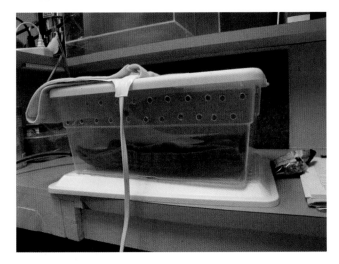

Figure 10.1 Recovery setup.

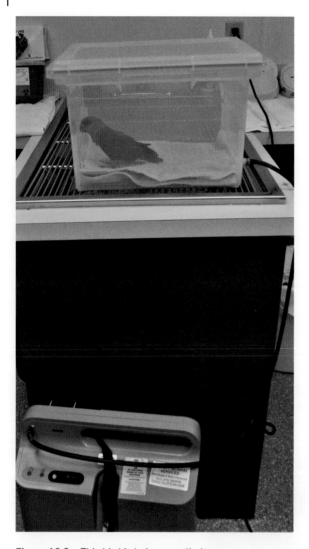

Figure 10.2 This bird is being supplied oxygen.

Technical Action

1) Restrain the bird in a towel and carry to the surgery suite.
2) Depending on the procedure and the surgeon's preference, the bird will have received pre-anesthetic analgesic/sedative combination.
3) The bird is placed on the warming system, sternal, while held in the towel, and induction of the anesthetic (injectable or mask inhalant) is begun.
4) When thoroughly relaxed, the bird should be intubated and secured.
5) Usually, the bird is now in dorsal recumbency, but it may depend on the surgery.
6) Monitoring equipment should be attached, and vital readings and recordings at intervals are initiated.

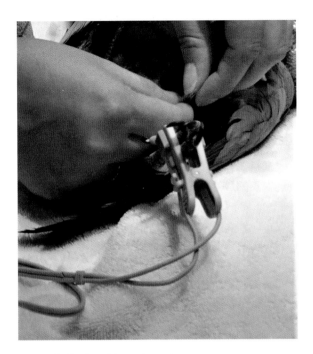

Figure 10.3 Attaching pulse oximetry.

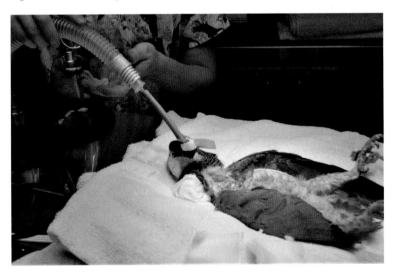

Figure 10.4 The endotracheal tube is in and taped. The bird is on a warming system.

7) The surgical site is swabbed with a surgical preparation solution. Take care not to excessively wet peripheral feathers. Local anesthesia may be administered to the surgical site, incision line, and/or lesion. Dab any bleeding dry, and swab the area three more times with the surgical scrub solution. Note: generally, alcohol is not used as it cools the bird. It can be used with caution for potential cooling. Swabbing the incision site with cotton swabs moistened with alcohol decreases the potential for cooling.

8) If feathers remain in the surgical site, it may be necessary to pluck them.
   a) Using sterile hemostats, clamp the base of the feather close to the skin.
   b) Pull the feather in the direction of the feather growth with a firm "pluck."
   c) Taken in the direction of growth minimizes damage to the follicle.
   d) Have a discussion with the owner prior to surgery that some feathers may need to be removed.
   e) Swab the area again after feather removal with the surgical scrub.
9) The surgeon/assistant should don a surgery gown, gloves, and open packs, including the drape.
10) Apply the drape.

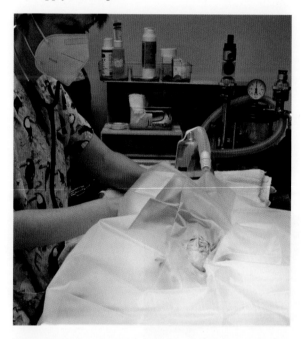

Figure 10.5 Plastic drapes are preferred as they can be cut to fit the incision area, are lightweight, and provide visualization of the bird under the drape. This can be useful so that the surgery can easily see respirations. The veterinary nurse has easy access to the bird for monitoring.

11) At some point during this preparation, the bird has entered a deep, surgical plane of anesthesia. If an inhalant agent is being used, dial back the concentration to maintenance.
12) Begin the surgery.
13) Following closure, the anesthesia will be discontinued. Keep the bird on plain oxygen until it starts to move. If using injectable agents, reverse those that can be reversed if necessary.
14) Extubate when the bird regains jaw tone and starts to move.
15) Remove the monitoring equipment as the bird begins to regain consciousness and moves.
16) When the bird is responding to touch and is trying to get away, the author covers and wraps a towel around the bird and places it in an incubator for recovery.
17) When the bird is awake, it will wriggle out of the towel and perch on it.
18) Depending on the procedure, additional medications may be administered.

19) A veterinary nurse or assistant should be assigned to the bird and be with it through the post-operative period until it is fully awake, ambulatory, and behaving normally. Even then, it is advisable to check on avian surgical patients at least every 10 minutes for several hours.

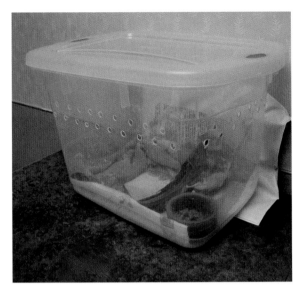

Figure 10.6 Hospital recovery cage, with heat and soft flooring. Recovery cages should provide security and comfort for the bird, but easy visibility for the veterinary team. Heat around the part of the cage allows the bird to choose where it is comfortable.

Rationale/Amplification

19: Postoperative observations must be planned, and preferably a staff person is assigned to stay with the bird. Postoperative support includes additional fluid therapy and analgesics administered at time intervals calculated from the initial analgesia. If the bird does not eat on its own within a couple of hours of recovery, it may need to be tube-fed. The advantage of gavage feeding of a concentrated nutritional formula ensures nutritional support.

BIBLIOGRAPHY

Speer BL. Basic anaesthesia. In: Chitty J, Monks L (eds). *BSAVA Manual of Avian Practice. A Foundation Manual.* 2018. BSAVA, Quedgeley, UK. pp 232–241.

11

Intubation

Birds have complete tracheal rings; therefore, endotracheal tubes are either non-cuffed, or if cuffed, the cuff is not inflated.

The trachea is usually 2.7 times longer and 1.3 times wider than that of a similar size/weight mammal.

The laryngeal structure is located at the base of the tongue, and the glottis is easily seen.

The glottis is connected to the distal syrinx via an elongated trachea.

The trachea divides into two primary bronchi at the syrinx.

The endotracheal tube should not extend completely to the syrinx.

Birds under 100 grams of weight are not as frequently intubated only because commercial tracheal tubes are not usually available: Modified tubes can be made from various catheters; however, with extremely small diameters, mucous plugs can occur.

Modified face masks can be used on smaller birds, if a fit so that respiration and anesthesia can be controlled.

Intubation allows for intermittent positive pressure ventilation using a small animal ventilator.

Intubation also allows for intratracheal medication to be administered, particularly in emergency situations.

Equipment

- Endotracheal tube (ET)
- Atraumatic forceps
- Tie (gauze, tape, length of ribbon or shoelace, etc.)
- Facemask (if for small animals, remove the rubber cuff)
- Towel for restraint

Technical Action

1) Select the endotracheal tube based on the bird's body weight and size.
2) Modify the face mask with a plastic wrap to allow a better seal. Cover the mask and then make a hole in the middle of the plastic with the forceps that the bird's head will be pushed through.
3) Sedate/induce the bird (if parenteral, use the mask with just oxygen; otherwise, with a sedated bird, use inhalant anesthesia): once relaxed and the beak can be easily opened, the tongue should be extended to visualize the glottis.

Manual of Clinical Procedures in Pet Birds, First Edition. Cathy A. Johnson-Delaney and Tracy Bennett.
© 2025 John Wiley & Sons, Inc. Published 2025 by John Wiley & Sons, Inc.
Companion website: www.wiley.com/go/johnson-delaney/manual

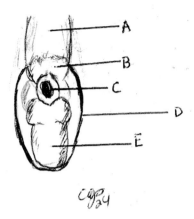

Figure 11.1 Diagram of the opened mouth with the upper beak at the top. A: Soft palate. B. Esophagus. C. Glottis. D. Lower beak. E. Tongue.

4) Extend the bird's neck so that the glottis and trachea are aligned with no neck flexion. This is usually done with an assistant holding and lifting the rhinotheca while supporting the back of the head.

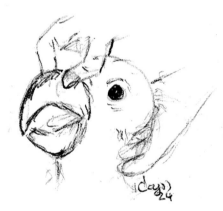

Figure 11.2 Opening the bird's beak. The rhinotheca (upper beak) is held by an assistant who is also supporting the back of the head.

5) Gently push down the lower beak (rhamphotheca) and pass the endotracheal tube into the trachea, leaving enough length to attach the tie material to secure it. It may be advisable to use a gauze sponge or syringe casing in the beak to prevent beak closure from compressing the tube.
6) Position the bird for the procedure and then connect the endotracheal tube to the machines to be used.

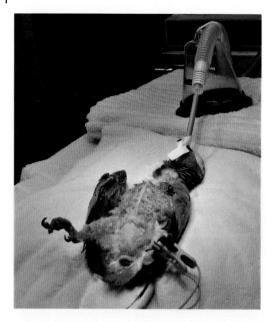

Figure 11.3 The tube is secured to the bird's beak. The tube is secured so that the angle is maintained. In this case, a larger mask worked to prop the tube/hose and a tape secured it.

7) The author prefers to have the connector fitting outside the mouth so that it can be easily connected to the anesthesia machine, ventilator, and capnograph. This also allows for quick disconnect if needed (especially on recovery).

8) Intermittent positive pressure ventilation should be done throughout anesthesia. This is usually done manually, although some small animal ventilators can be set and used in avian anesthesia (IPPV).

Rationale/Amplification

Intubation is preferred during any anesthesia.
   a) Prevents potential aspiration.
   b) Provides a reliable airway.
Endotracheal tubes are available in many sizes.
Face masks suitable for small mammals can be used; however, the rubber fitting ring is usually removed. A cut surgical glove or piece of plastic wrap can be used to provide a seal around the neck of the bird and is customized per patient. (The rubber ring orifice is usually too large to seal around the bird's neck, and as the bird is anesthetized, it often will grab the rubber ring orifice and damage it and the mask itself).
Masks can be made of syringe containers/casings, small tubes, and even connector fittings – depending on the bird size/weight and beak/head shape.
IPPV counters decreased respiration, decreased tidal volume, and decreased patient oxygenation during anesthesia.
Remember that the gas entering the bird through the endotracheal tube will cool the bird. Maintenance of body temperature is critical during anesthesia and surgery.

BIBLIOGRAPHY

Greenacre CB, Gerhardt L. Psittacine and passerine birds. In: Ballard B, Cheek R (eds). *Exotic Animal Medicine for the Veterinary Technician*. Third Edition. 2017. Wiley Blackwell, Ames, IA. pp 100–142.

Montesinos A. Basic techniques. In: Chitty J, Monks D (eds). *BSAVA Manual of Avian Practice. A Foundation Manual*. 2018. BSAVA, Quedgeley, UK. pp 216–2410.

12

Gavage and Lavage

- Delivery of medications and/or fluids directly into the crop eliminates the problems of voluntarily swallowing by the bird and allows the clinician to administer an accurate dosage.
- Entering the crop via a tube allows for aspiration of the material for microbiology and cytology testing. This material more accurately represents the condition of the crop and even that of the gastrointestinal tract.
- During times when the ingesta is not exiting the crop due to generalized gastrointestinal disease and stasis, passage of a tube allows for aspiration and removal of food and material.
- Passage of a tube also allows for placement of isotonic fluids for fluid therapy directly into the crop.
- Lavage may be done following removal of the material – this may also remove irritants or pathogens.
- Prior to administering nutrition into the crop, the bird should be adequately hydrated, and must not vomit or regurgitate.

Procedure Collection of Diagnostic Materials

Collection of microbiological or cytological materials

Technical Action

1) Restrain the bird usually using a towel. Hold the bird in an upright position.
2) The examiner should use a speculum or have an additional person use a gauze bandage material to hold the beak open.

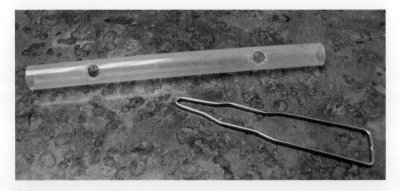

Figure 12.1 Types of oral speculums that can be used to hold a beak open.

Manual of Clinical Procedures in Pet Birds, First Edition. Cathy A. Johnson-Delaney and Tracy Bennett.
© 2025 John Wiley & Sons, Inc. Published 2025 by John Wiley & Sons, Inc.
Companion website: www.wiley.com/go/johnson-delaney/manual

3) In birds with weight less than 200 grams, a culture-type swab or sterile swab can be passed directly into the crop for a swab of material.
4) In larger birds, it is usually necessary to pass a sterile metal crop needle or sterile tubing attached to a sterile syringe for material aspiration.
   a) The material from the needle or tubing can be dropped onto glass slides for immediate cytology or dried for staining or cytological examination.
   b) The material can also be submitted for bacterial and/or fungal culture or sent for PCR or next-generation PCR screening.

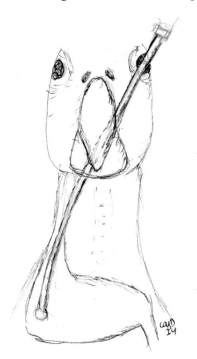

Figure 12.2 The feeding needle/stomach tube is passed from the bird's left side of the open mouth, back and to the right, and passed down the neck into the crop. The tube can easily be felt passing down the neck and placement confirmed by feeling the end of the tube inside the crop through the skin just above the sternum.

Procedure Crop Wash

1) Nonbacteriostatic fluid may be injected into a crop and massaged to mix with crop materials.
2) This can then be aspirated and submitted for microbiology and cytology testing.
3) It is useful particularly if there have been impacted dry materials palpated within the crop or in cases where the material is beginning to ferment within the crop due to gastrointestinal hypomotility.
4) If the bird has ingested toxic materials and foreign bodies: aspiration of such agents and then introducing more fluids to further aspirate the materials may be a first step to decrease toxin absorption.
5) A wash is simply installing fluids: and it may serve to soothe the crop.

Technical Action

1) Restrain the bird as given above.
2) Pass a crop tube into the crop and inject a small volume of nonbacteriostatic fluid.
3) Massage the crop.
4) Aspirate the materials and liquid out of the crop.
5) After removal of the fluid, a medication can then be injected into the crop and the tube withdrawn.

Rationale/Amplification

Note: in any bird that is regurgitating or vomiting, prior to any additional of fluids to the crop, the bird should be intubated. This requires sedation and/or anesthesia. This is necessary to prevent accidental aspiration.

Procedure Gavage Feeding via Crop Tube

1) Indications are to provide nutrition and fluids in birds that are severely anorectic and/or dehydrated.
2) The direct volume of a feeding solution and/or fluids can be calculated based on calories and fluids needed as per that body weight.
3) Quickly passing a tube and instilling materials into the crop can be far less stressful to the bird than trying to hand-feed it and place fluids directly into the mouth.

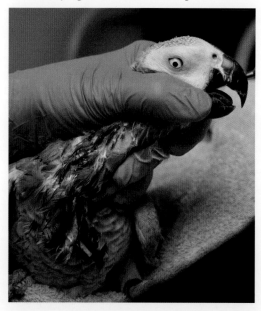

4) Several formulations of solutions containing a source of quick calories, protein, vitamins, and minerals are commercially available. All of these come with dosage per body weight guidelines, as well as indications for usage.
5) Crop capacity estimates: 30–50 mL/kg body weight. In ill birds, consider using a volume of 20 mL/kg. This can be administered multiple times a day, depending on the medication, feeding formula, illness, and crop emptying time.

Technical Action

1) Restrain the bird and hold upright.
2) In birds reluctant to open their mouths, another staff person may be necessary to retract the beak using a gauze bandage.
3) If an oral speculum is used, it needs to be one that does not cause trauma to the beak lateral walls.
4) Premeasure the tube by holding it up, alongside the bird, and determining how far it is to be inserted to reach the caudoventral border of the crop.
5) The solution to be administered should be warmed to avian body temperature.
6) Lubricate the tube with a small amount of neutral gel or even a little warm water.
7) With the bird held with the mouth open, the administrator can easily pass the tube from the right side of the mouth over the tongue and down the side of the esophagus that lies against the lateral left wall of the neck. In many birds, you can see or feel the tube sliding down to the crop.
8) Palpate the end of the feeding tube within the crop.
9) Attach the syringe with the warmed feeding liquid and slowly start to inject it into the crop. As you see the fluid fill the crop, you can increase the speed of the injection.
10) When the syringe is empty, quickly withdraw the tube and remove the speculum.
11) If a collapsible tube was used, prior to withdrawal, crimp it off at the syringe tip. This will prevent the material from dripping from the tube to possibly leak near the pharynx and cause coughing or even aspiration

Rationale/Amplification

For medicating and administering nutrition and even oral fluids to the severely ill patient, crop tube gavage is the quickest and most efficacious way to administer substances per os. It is quick and usually minimally stressful.
The volume of food or medication is largely dependent on the size of the bird.
Passerines may not have very well-developed pouches, unlike psittacines. Plan to administer slightly smaller volumes than you would to a psittacine of that body weight (Table 12.1).

Table 12.1   Suggested volumes and frequency of gavage feeding in anorectic birds. Generally, use a volume of 3–5% of body weight in milliliters.

Species	Volume (mL)	Frequency
Canary, finch	0.1–0.5	Q 4 h
Budgerigar	0.5–3	Q 6 h
Lovebird	1–3	Q 6 h
Cockatiel	1–8	Q 6 h
Conure (small)	3–12	Q 6 h
Conure (large)	7–24	Q 6–8 h
Amazon African grey	5–35	Q 8 h
Cockatoo	10–40	Q 8–12 h
Macaw	20–60	Q 8–12 h

Source: Guzman et al. (2023)/with permission of Elsevier.

BIBLIOGRAPHY

Guzman DS-M, Beaufrere H, Welle KR, Heatley J, Visser M, Harms CA. Birds. In: Carpenter JW, Harms CA (eds). *Carpenter's Exotic Animal Formulary*. Sixth Edition. 2023. Elsevier, St. Louis, MO. pp 222–444.

Montesinos A. Basic techniques. In: Chitty J, Monks D (eds). *BSAVA Manual of Avian Practice. A Foundation Manual*. 2018. British Small Animal Veterinary Association, Quedgeley, UK. pp 215–231.

13

Coelomocentesis

Procedure

Coelomocentesis is the technique of removing free fluid from the coelomic cavity of the bird. Because of avian anatomy, fluid from an organ, and neoplasia, hemorrhage will occur in the coelom, and be restricted by the presence of air sacs. The abdominal wall may be visibly distended and in some cases discolored (hemocoelom, egg yolk material, free ingesta from gastrointestinal rupture, etc.). The bird may present with dyspnea due to impedance of action of the respiratory bellows. The bird may have a pendulous abdomen that restricts normal posture and cloacal clearance – the tail feathers may appear pasted and/or the material may accumulate on the vent.

Due to the avian anatomy, it is advisable to try and visualize the fluid rather than just aspirate – there is very little free space within a bird as compared to a mammal, and it is possible to penetrate an organ or air sac.

Visualization can be done with ultrasonography (preferably) and with transillumination using a very bright source such as a Finoff transilluminator or the light source of an endoscope.

Considering that penetrating the coelom is likely painful, it is recommended that the bird be administered a sedative with an analgesic. Once the fluid is removed, depending on the cause and the fluid, proceeding to full anesthesia for surgery is an option.

Any bird with abdominal distention expected to have free fluid should be kept in an upright position to not compromise the lungs and keep the fluid at the most ventral area.

Purpose

To remove the fluid from the coelomic cavity.

Equipment

- Analgesics/sedatives (see Chapter 24)
- Oxygen, mask
- Blood pressure cuff, Doppler
- ECG and other surgical monitoring equipment
- Towel for restraint
- Warmed environment for post-procedure recovery
- Diagnostic collection tubes and microscopic slides
- Ultrasound machine and/or transilluminator
- Ultrasound gel and alcohol

Manual of Clinical Procedures in Pet Birds, First Edition. Cathy A. Johnson-Delancy and Tracy Bennett.
© 2025 John Wiley & Sons, Inc. Published 2025 by John Wiley & Sons, Inc.
Companion website: www.wiley.com/go/johnson-delaney/manual

- Surgical preparation solution
- 25–23 ga butterfly infusion catheter needles and syringes
- Gauze sponges
- Topical anesthetic cream
- Warm water, cotton, and towels to clean the vent and tail.

Technical Action

1) Restrain the bird, by holding it upright.
2) For initial assessment, wet the feathers with a surgical solution or ultrasound gel so that the skin and distention are visualized.
3) The author's preference is to use ultrasound images to visualize the fluid and fluid volume.
4) Administer the analgesic/sedative and initiate oxygen flow. This procedure is usually done with the bird conscious.
5) Prepare the area to be entered: apply a small amount of anesthetic cream to the area.
6) While the bird is becoming sedated, further push back the feathers and gently swab/cleanse the area with a surgical preparation solution, including removing any fecal/urate pasting of the vent and tail.
7) When the bird is relaxed, using ultrasonography (a small amount of alcohol on skin) or transillumination, visualize the fluid.

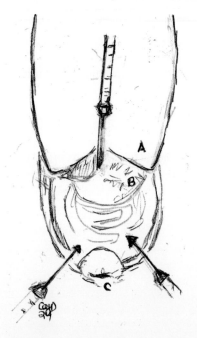

Figure 13.1 Three potential sites for coelomic centesis depending on where the fluid has collected and organ size and placement. It is advisable to use ultrasound guidance to insert the needle and observe fluid and organ movement. A: Sternum. B: Ventriculus. C: Vent.

8) Insert the needle just into the fluid, and either let it drip through the tube into a collection tube or very gently and slowly aspirate the fluid. The bird's respiration should be watched closely during this process as fluid withdrawal should make respiration deeper and easier. However, be aware that if there is a space-occupying a mass as part of the distention, there may have be

vascular compromise as well, and the if vital parameters change (like blood pressure and ECG), you may want to cease removal of the fluid until the cardiovascular system has equalized.

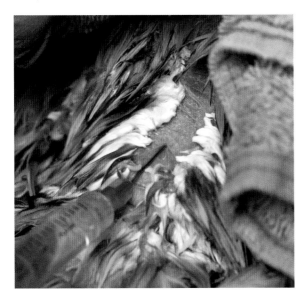

9) If frank blood is seen during the procedure, stop immediately. Check with visualizing as much as possible to determine if an organ or vascular structure was penetrated or if this is actually what the fluid is.
10) Wipe off any remaining gel, alcohol, oozing fluid, or vent/tail soiling.
11) In many cases, the bird is returned to a warmed environment for recovery, while the fluid is tested, and a diagnostic plan is formulated.

Rationale/Amplification

7: Ultrasonography is useful to determine if there is a mass, potential retained egg, organomegaly, and even may hint at the composition of the fluid – purely anechoic is likely effusion, while the egg yolk is dense and particulate, and blood can have almost a grainy–flaky look to it.

8: The needle will be visible on insertion and then can be directed at the largest accumulation of the fluid. Structures can be avoided by doing ultrasound-guided centesis. Fluid testing includes culture, cytology, and specific gravity as is done in other animals.

11: Let the owner know what the fluid appears to be and how that affects the diagnostic/treatment plan. Let the owner know that there may be bruising of the abdominal wall where the needle went in, but this should be minor. Also, let the owner know if the abdominal wall is now slightly loose as the appearance may be alarming, especially if there was some feather loss over what had been a bulging lower body.

BIBLIOGRAPHY

Campbell TW. Cytology. In: Richie BW, Harrison GJ, Harrison LR (eds). *Avian Medicine: Principles and Application*. 1994. Wingers Publishing Inc., Lake Worth, FL.

14

Nebulization

Purpose

1) To assist as an expectorant and/or a way to hydrate mucous membranes.
2) Adjunctive therapy for upper and/or lower respiratory disease.
3) To introduce antimicrobials directly into non-granulomatous diseased airways (nebulized particles cannot penetrate avian granulomas (usually)).

Equipment

- A jet-type nebulizer (rather than an ultrasonic one) that produces smaller droplets that likely will have better penetration of the airways, particularly the lower airways. These are sold for human use. Buy the model that will produce the smaller droplet/particle size.
- Extension tubes and hoses (usually come with the nebulizer).
- A chamber for use: can be constructed from a plastic storage container-type bin, with holes in the side to accommodate the insertion of the tube from the nebulizing chamber.
- Sterile saline, syringes/needles for measuring agents for the nebulizing chamber. Most chambers hold 5–7 mL, and the nebulizer will complete the expulsion usually within 15–20 minutes.
- Oxygen through a regulator can be used instead of room air through the nebulizer.

Technical Action

1) Mix a nebulizing solution.
2) Fill the nebulizer chamber, and attach the hose to the chamber.
3) Place the bird within the chamber, preferably on a low perch or small towel for comfortable footing

Manual of Clinical Procedures in Pet Birds, First Edition. Cathy A. Johnson-Delaney and Tracy Bennett.
© 2025 John Wiley & Sons, Inc. Published 2025 by John Wiley & Sons, Inc.
Companion website: www.wiley.com/go/johnson-delaney/manual

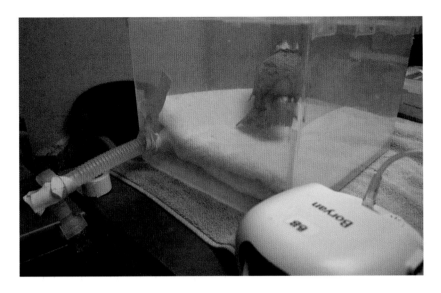

4) Start the nebulizer and have someone observe during the entire process.
5) If the bird is nervous at the start of the vapor entering the chamber, dim the lights as this may have a calming effect. Also, talk to the bird to calm it.
6) If a bird is greatly distressed at the start, a mild sedative can be given such as nasal midazolam prior to nebulizing. Once the bird has calmed, it may be replaced in the chamber, and the process starts.

Rationale/Amplification

\# Agents used must be nonirritant and nontoxic to both the bird and the personnel since the personnel will be exposed to the agents upon release of the bird from the chamber.
\# Potentially effective antimicrobial agents should be chosen: consult a current avian formulary.
\# Constructing a chamber using a commercial storage bin allows visualization of the bird during the process and can easily be disinfected. They are also inexpensive.
\# Frequency of nebulization and duration of treatment depend on the disease being treated and response.
\# Owners can continue this treatment at home: clinics may have nebulizers and chambers to loan to clients. Pre-made nebulizing solutions can be dispensed as a prescription.

BASIC NEBULIZING FORMULAS FOR USE IN BIRDS

1) F10 SC 1:250 dilution with sterile saline or sterile water.
2) *N*-acetyl-L-cysteine (10–20%) – mix to achieve a concentration of 22 mg/mL in sterile water.
3) Aminophylline – mix to achieve a concentration of 3 mg/mL in sterile water or a sufficient volume of saline to run for 15 minutes.
4) Hypertonic saline (3%) (has mucolytic properties).
5) Physiologic saline (0.9%) – hydrate mucous membranes.

BIBLIOGRAPHY

Chitty J, Monks D. Lower respiratory tract disease. In: Chitty J, Monks D (eds). *BSAVA Manual of Avian Practice. A Foundation Manual*. 2018. British Small Animal Veterinary Association, Quedgeley, UK. pp 324–333.

Guzman DS-M, Beaufrere H, Welle KR, Heatley J, Visser M, Harms CA. Birds. In: Carpenter JW, Harms CA (eds). *Carpenter's Exotic Animal Formulary*. Sixth Edition. 2023. Elsevier, St. Louis, MO. pp 222–444.

15

Egg Retention Procedures

Egg retention is often called "egg binding," but technically, it should be referred to as post-ovulatory stasis or delayed oviposition. It is a failure of an egg to pass normally through the oviduct. It equates with dystocia in mammals.

There can be many underlying causes, and egg retention is often multifactorial. Contributing factors can include nutritional deficiencies, especially calcium (complicated by lack of UVB light and vitamin D3 deficiency); mechanical obstruction in the oviduct or cloaca; smooth muscle functional deficiencies of the oviduct and/or uterus; damage including tears; infection and inflammation of the oviduct; obesity; poor abdominal muscles from lack of exercise; and improper husbandry including inadequate housing and nesting conditions. Some species that may lay excessively have fatigue of the oviduct, and the egg fails to move and is expelled.

When presented, a full history needs to be provided, and the bird should be observed in the cage. Usually, the bird has an abnormal posture, often with the tail and rump elevated, and the bird is leaning forward. She may be on the bottom of the cage. Other acute clinical signs include depression, dyspnea, ruffled feathers, and an enlarged ventral coelom (abdomen). The bird may be straining with the vent pulsing and leaking urates, urine, and feces. Larger birds may show paresis of the legs or lameness.

Procedure

Examination and preparation for egg evacuation

Purpose

To support the bird physically during the examination and diagnostic process to determine the extent of egg retention, position, and condition of the egg.

Complications

- History of poor diet (primarily of seeds – likely calcium and protein deficiency), lack of vitamin D3 (UVB light exposure), age of the bird, and stage of the egg laying process.
- Any underlying disease, especially infection or inflammation of the reproductive tract.
- Duration of the retained egg(s) and physical status of the bird (i.e. fluffed, on the bottom of the cage, and dyspneic)

Manual of Clinical Procedures in Pet Birds, First Edition. Cathy A. Johnson-Delaney and Tracy Bennett.
© 2025 John Wiley & Sons, Inc. Published 2025 by John Wiley & Sons, Inc.
Companion website: www.wiley.com/go/johnson-delaney/manual

- Prolapse of the cloaca, vagina, uterus, or oviduct due to chronic straining. If the tissues are not dried or damaged, with correction of egg retention, tissues may be replaced and surgically corrected and sutured. In cases of a damaged reproductive tract, excision of tissue and/or hysterectomy may be needed. That technique is beyond the scope of this book.
- Egg-related peritonitis due to egg yolk material in the coelom. It can be septic or nonseptic. This can be detected with ultrasonography.
- Coelomic herniation. This will require surgical correction once the retained egg(s) are removed. The surgical procedure is beyond the scope of this book.

Equipment

- Supportive environmental equipment such as an incubator, oxygen provision, and warming systems.
- Fluids such as a 50:50 mix of saline and 5% dextrose, warmed, appropriate delivery needles, catheters, and syringes.
- Calcium gluconate for injection (100 mg/kg SC into the fluid pocket)
- Scale
- Ultrasound system
- Radiology capability
- Restraint equipment including towels.
- Analgesics: such as an opioid, NSAID, and needle/syringes. (e.g. butorphanol at 1–2 mg/kg IM)
- Topical analgesic/anesthetic such as 1% lidocaine to irrigate the cloaca.
- Anxiolytic/muscle relaxant such as a benzodiazepine (midazolam at 0.1–0.5 mg/kg SC or IM) and reversal by flumazenil injection if desired
- Warmed saline for irrigation of the cloaca
- Crop feeding tube and supportive emergency formulation (such as EmerAid® and Lafeber Co.)

Technical Action

1) Weigh the bird.
2) Physical examination including palpation and auscultation.
3) The author assumes some level of pain associated with this condition. Administration of an analgesic along with an anxiolytic/relaxant will facilitate imaging and further diagnostics and treatment.
4) Imaging (this may be delayed until after fluids, tube feeding, and stabilization): traditionally started with lateral and VD views. If dyspnea, oxygen supplementation is suggested.
5) Ultrasonography of the abdomen (coelom). This will image the number of eggs and the condition of any eggs or follicles. Take care during the process to hold the bird in an upright position and put minimal pressure on the abdomen. This can often be done quickly during the initial physical examination.

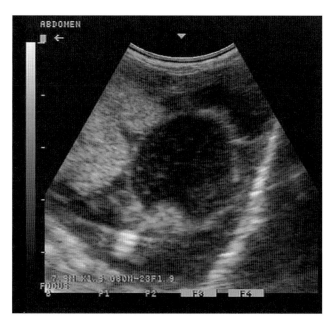

Figure 15.1 Ultrasound picture of the retained egg. This egg has a calcified shell.

6) Depending on findings, full bloodwork may be considered and drawn.
7) Administer SC fluids at a dose of 25–50 mL/kg; administer calcium gluconate into the SC fluids for slow absorption. Administer a small meal into the crop via a feeding tube.
8) Place the bird in the controlled supportive caging and allow for fluid absorption at least 15–20 minutes before further handling and manipulation.

Rationale/Amplification

3,7,8. These steps are crucial to aiding the bird to be able to correct deficiencies and, in many cases, these alone will allow the egg to be laid.
5. Ultrasonography using a point-of-care system can be done very quickly and does not seem to be stressful to the bird. A small amount of alcohol to part the feathers if needed, and only a tiny bit of gel is needed to observe the eggs/follicles, detect free fluid in the coelom, and even image the heart. This information greatly determines the course of treatment.

Procedure

Topical application of prostaglandin

Purpose

Medically cause propulsion of the egg by using topical prostaglandin E2 or dinoprostone gel. This should only be done if the bird is in good condition, the uterus is intact, deemed disease-free, and is nonneoplastic. The egg also cannot be adhered to the oviduct, misshapen or oversized.

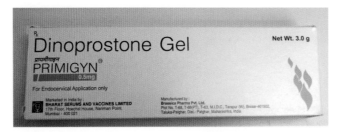

Figure 15.2 Source: Bharat Serums and Vaccines Limited (BSV).

Complications

- If the above conditions are not met, it could cause severe distress, uterine rupture, egg rupture, and compromise to the cardiovascular system due to the straining.
- *Note*: oxytocin is no longer routinely used in birds as it does not work well to expulse the egg and may compromise the cardiovascular system.

Equipment

- Prostaglandin E2 or dinoprostone gel
- Bird previously treated with the above supportive care and is housed in a supportive environment such as an incubator.
- Towel for restraint
- Procedure gloves as protection from touching this gel.

Technical Action

1) Put on protective gloves.
2) Hold the bird in the towel so that the cloaca is accessible.
3) Place 1 mL/kg body weight of the gel in the cloaca (can be done using a small syringe).
4) Place the bird back in the supportive housing and observe.
5) The egg is usually expelled within 15 minutes. Contractions will be visible.

Rationale/Amplification

3. This volume has proven effective.
5. If the egg is not expelled, then manual expression may be tried.

Procedure

Manual delivery of the egg

Purpose

To manually manipulate an egg within the distal oviduct to exit the cloaca. This is usually only tried if a. the prostaglandin failed, or b. there is a reason not to use prostaglandins (such as the bird not determined to be in strong physical condition, or c. there may be concurrent reproductive tract disease.

Complications

- Pressure on the bird's abdomen may be uncomfortable. This procedure is usually done under general anesthesia.
- If the egg is thickened or too large to pass through the uterine opening, ovocentesis may be needed.
- The egg could crack and collapse, leaving the shell and material within the oviduct.
- Excessive manipulation can damage the oviduct and/or cloacal tissues.

Equipment

- Butorphanol (2 mg/kg IM)
- Inhalant anesthesia, machine, and mask delivery system (such as isoflurane)
- Sterile lubricant (such as KY® jelly)
- Cotton-tipped applicators
- Atraumatic vascular forceps
- Warmed saline in a syringe for irrigation
- Gauze sponges and towels to remove excess gel for cleanup.
- Warming pad and monitoring equipment used during inhalant general anesthesia.
- Syringe (1–5 cc depending on size of the egg) and needle (usually 18–22 ga) for ovocentesis if necessary.

Technical Action

1) After supportive care of fluids, calcium, and feeding and the bird appears stable, remove the bird from the incubator and administer additional butorphanol if it has been more than 4 hours since the original butorphanol/midazolam administration.
2) After at least 15 minutes, the bird can be masked with oxygen and inhalant anesthesia and attached to the monitoring equipment.
3) The bird should be placed in dorsal recumbency on a slanted platform to keep the head and body elevated.
4) Lubricate the cloaca with a small amount of a sterile lubricant. The uterine opening can be slightly dilated with a lubricated cotton-tipped applicator.

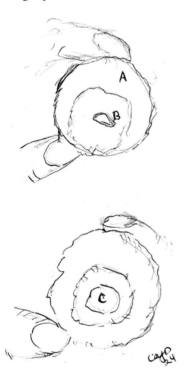

Figure 15.3 Manual gentle pressure on the exterior of the vent, as the cloacal tissue prolapses slightly. The vent and inside of the cloaca should be lubricated before beginning to put pressure. A. Prolapsing cloacal tissue. B. Uterine opening. C. Egg showing through the opening.

5) Palpate the egg through the body wall and apply a constant, gentle digital pressure on the proximal part of the egg to push it toward the cloaca.
6) Continue as the egg becomes visible. Additional gel may be needed during the expulsion.
7) If the egg is thickened or deemed too large to pass through the vaginal opening without causing damage or prolapse, ovocentesis can be done.
8) With the egg visible in the vaginal opening, insert a needle (usually 22–23 ga but depends on the size of the), into the egg and aspirate the contents. With gentle digital pressure, collapse the egg.
9) With continued gentle pressure, manually push the collapsed egg out of the vaginal opening. Irrigate with saline as necessary. If there are egg fragments, remove these using the atraumatic vascular forceps, taking care not to damage any mucosa.
10) Irrigate the cloaca well to remove all egg remnants.
11) Dry the tail feathers and ventrum with towels.

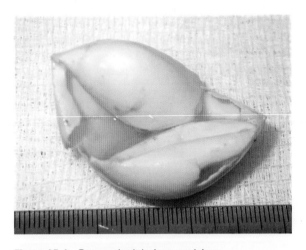

Figure 15.4 Egg crushed during expulsion.

Rationale/Amplification

4: The sterile lubricant should be warmed, as should saline used for irrigation.

7: A soft egg may be difficult to push toward the vaginal opening. Older texts suggest transcoelomic ovocentesis of the egg, so it can then pass on its own. However, there is a great risk of causing secondary coelomitis due to leakage of egg contents or damage to the uterus/oviduct. This is no longer recommended. In the author's experience, soft eggs can be gently manipulated just as hardened eggs.

8: If the egg cannot be passed, surgical intervention is required, which is beyond the scope of this book.

BIBLIOGRAPHY

Curd S. Egg retention. In: Chitty J, Monks D (eds). *BSAVA Manual of Avian Practice. A Foundation Manual.* 2018. British Small Animal Veterinary Association, Quedgeley, UK. pp 350–357.

Wyre N. Psittacines. In: Graham JE, Doss GA, Beaufrere H (eds). *Exotic Animal Emergency and Critical Care Medicine.* 2021. John Wiley & Sons, Inc., Hoboken, NJ. pp 1491–1550.

16

Cardiac Procedures

Cardiac disease is common in pet birds. Many are still fed diets largely composed of seeds and nuts that are high in fat and lack many other nutrients. Pet birds usually get little exercise, in contrast to their wild counterparts. Unfortunately, obesity is common, as is atherosclerosis. Complete cardiac examinations should be incorporated into regular avian examinations, particularly as birds age and have a history of a seed-based diet. Blood evaluations should include triglycerides, which can be elevated with atherosclerosis. No one test definitively diagnoses cardiovascular disease, but serial examinations and recording trends can help plan a program of management, prevention, and treatment if the disease is already present.

The regular physical examination can give impressions of general perfusion – poor oxygenation and perfusion may be manifested with cool feet and bluish nail vessel if visible, bluish tint to mucosa, facial skin (macaws), and dyspnea with a small amount of exertion (exercise intolerance), although primary respiratory disease should also be ruled out.

The initial examination is done with the stethoscope, placed over the sternum in multiple areas, as well as over the back. Arrhythmias and murmurs may be found, although not fully characterized just with auscultation.

Regular radiographs, lateral and ventrodorsal (VD) may give impressions of cardiac size and great vessel density including any calcifications, but do not definitely diagnose what type of cardiovascular disease is present.

Manual of Clinical Procedures in Pet Birds, First Edition. Cathy A. Johnson-Delaney and Tracy Bennett.
© 2025 John Wiley & Sons, Inc. Published 2025 by John Wiley & Sons, Inc.
Companion website: www.wiley.com/go/johnson-delaney/manual

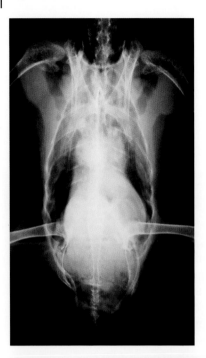

Figure 16.1 VD radiograph. Appearance of a cardiac silhouette. Please note that this bird has several abnormalities, including an enlarged heart.

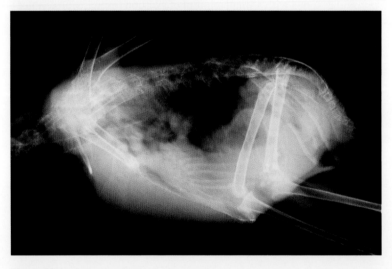

Figure 16.2 Lateral radiograph showing heart and great vessels. Heart size on radiographs does not provide diagnosis of heart disease or the type of heart disease, only size and perhaps density. More diagnostic tests are needed.

To better examine the cardiovascular system, three additional tests are of value, although interpretation of the electrocardiograph (ECG) and echocardiograph is beyond the scope of this text.

Depending on the temperament and clinical condition of the bird, prolonged restraint and manipulation for obtaining the ECG, blood pressure, and echocardiograph may cause distress. Light sedation with a benzodiazepine such as midazolam will not interfere with the tests and will decrease the stress. The dosage of the sedative will depend on the species, but in general, most birds will calm with 2 mg/kg delivered intranasally. It can be reversed with flumazenil given by intramuscular (IM) injection.

Equipment used for cardiac measurements in birds needs to be able to read higher heart rates. Older machines designed primarily for dogs and cats do not measure heart rates above 250 bpm. Newer equipment can accurately read the parameters. The types of electrodes for use in birds need to be smaller and atraumatic. Alligator-type clips used in mammals may damage the skin. Because bird skin is thin, for smaller birds, 25-gauge hypodermic needles wetted with alcohol may work. Larger birds can have adhesive–electrode patches, although they need to be applied directly to the skin, and occasionally some body feathers may need to be plucked. One company has electrodes that are loops that can be fastened around a limb, and a small dab of contact gel applied provides totally atraumatic leads. Ideally, there should be four electrodes placed, but the authors use the three-loop lead system and record diagnostic ECGs even in birds as small as canaries.

Procedure

Electrocardiographic recording and/or monitoring

Purpose

To obtain a diagnostic ECG and/or continually monitor the heart during a procedure. The ECG is valuable to characterize arrythmias, electrolyte imbalances, electrical axis, dilation, etc.

Complications

- The machine must be capable of accurately detecting the electrical activity of hearts with rates above 250 bpm. It should be able to detect very low electrical transmission.
- The interpretive software or paper print-out must be adjustable to provide traces of diagnostic quality that measurements can be made.
- Some electrodes are clips that may traumatize the avian thin skin, and others for small animals may be too large to position on a bird's body.
- Avian hearts depolarize from the epicardium to the endocardium, so the QRS complex appears inverted compared to a mammalian trace.
- The bird needs to be relatively still to get a diagnostic trace.

Equipment

- Restraint equipment (e.g. towels and restraint strap)
- Isopropyl alcohol
- Electrode contact gel
- Anesthetic cream (if using clips, especially with teeth)
- Gauze sponges
- ECG machine, attachments for the computer, and electrodes (whatever type recommended for use with that machine)
- Software for recording, measuring, and evaluating.
- Some machines still print directly on a strip – then strip paper, and ink is also required.
- Sedative (some birds consider Intranasal midazolam at 2 mg/kg)

Technical Action

1) Restrain the bird, usually held in an upright normal posture. A small amount of water or alcohol may be needed to part the feathers for the attachment of the electrodes.

2) If using clips, apply a small amount of anesthetic cream where the clips are to be attached and allow it to be in contact for several minutes before attaching clips. If using a hypodermic needle that the clip will attach to, again use the anesthetic cream, and wait for several minutes before inserting the needles. If using loops, be sure they are snug and in contact with the skin, but not so tight as to cut off circulation. Instead of passing the wing through a loop, wet a small area of the skin in the right axilla to part the feathers, place the loop against the skin, add a dab of the electrode gel, and then using a nonadhesive wrap, secure the loop in the axilla.

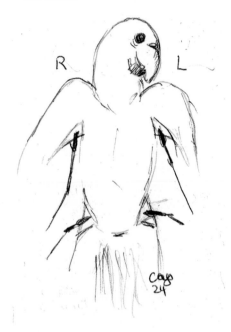

Figure 16.3 Placement sites for needle or clip-type electrode systems. A small amount of alcohol is needed to part the feathers over the wing axillary skin and use the skin from the body to the legs. Small needles can be used, and then the clips are attached to them, or small, atraumatic clips can be used to attach to these skin-web areas.

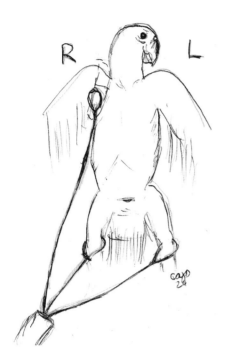

Figure 16.4 Placement positions for the 3-lead loop electrode system. Loops are cinched snuggly to prevent slipping, but not so tight to occlude blood flow. A little bit of alcohol is used to part the feathers, and a small amount of electrode gel is used on the cables for contact. The legs are inserted through the loops. The right axillary loop is placed in the axilla – part the feathers with a little alcohol, apply a dab of gel to the loop, and fix it into the axilla using a stretchy, nonstick bandage material to hold it in place against the skin.

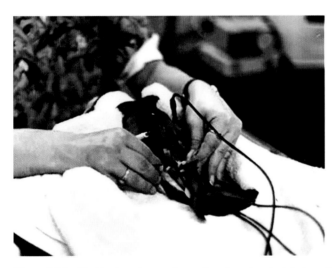

Figure 16.5 Bird in dorsal recumbency, towel, and restraint strap. 4-lead ECG recorder.

1) Attach the electrodes to the needles or clips. Usually, these are color-coded/labeled. The loops already color-coded and attached to the ECG machine. A small amount of alcohol may be needed to part the feathers and aid in contact. A small amount of contact gel may be needed with some types of electrodes.

2) If the bird is wiggling against the restraint, a sedative can be given prior to attaching the electrodes. If the bird starts resisting once the electrodes are placed, then administer the sedative. Usually IN midazolam begins to have action within 3–5 minutes.

3) When a steady trace is viewed, begin the recording for diagnostic purposes. Run the trace for several minutes to get a good characterization of the cardiac rhythm.

4) Save the recording. Make a printout if the setup will do that. An extra trace strip is nice to give to the owner.

5) Remove the electrodes and dry the feathers with a gauze and the towel.

6) If no other diagnostic testing is needed with a sedated bird, flumazenil can be given to reverse the midazolam. Most species can be given 0.05–0.1 mg/kg IN or IM.

7) Return the bird to its home cage, gently unwrapping it from the towel.

Rationale/Amplification

4: Sometimes, the order of sedation versus attaching electrodes may be reversed – it depends on how the bird adjusts to being restrained. The sedative will not affect the cardiac analysis.

5: Optimally allow 2–3 minutes of tracing to be viewed and recorded. The author turns off the audible "beep" that marks QRS waves or arrythmias as this sound may agitate the bird.

6. Once recorded, measurements and assessments can be made for diagnosis. Interpretation is beyond the scope of this text. Do note that the S-wave will be negative due to avian heart depolarization from the exterior to the interior of the myocardium.

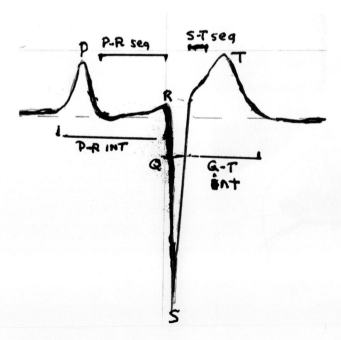

Figure 16.6 Avian ECG Trace.

Procedure

Blood pressure (BP) trend monitoring

Purpose

To use the indirect method of assessing blood pressure trends using an audio Doppler, inflatable cuff, and sphygmomanometer on a wing or leg.

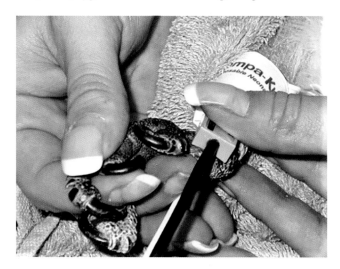

Figure 16.7 Blood pressure on the tibial–tarsal artery.

Wing:

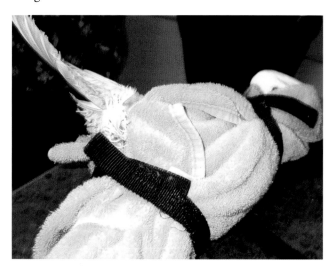

Figure 16.8 Positioning for wing extension. If the bird struggles, light sedation may be necessary. The author rarely sedates for blood pressure checks, either on the wing or the leg.

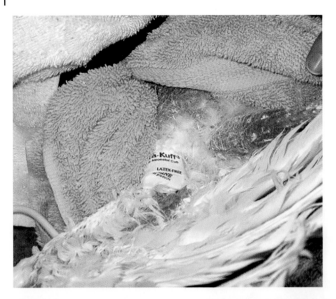

Figure 16.9   Placement of the cuff close to the body. Use the appropriate sized pediatric cuff as marked on the cuff itself.

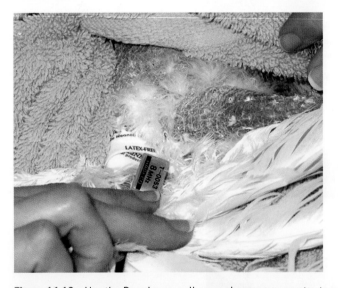

Figure 16.10   Use the Doppler as well as a sphygmomanometer to monitor systolic blood pressure.

Complications

- Even the smallest (neonatal) commercial cuffs may be too large for birds less than 150 grams, thereby rendering measurements useless.
- Because only the systolic beat is used to measure the upper limit of blood pressure, the diastolic beat is not assessed. This does allow trends to be noted, which are especially useful during surgeries, rehydration, and to monitor hypertension treatments.
- A stressed, painful, or struggling bird may have an elevated blood pressure. An anemic, cardiovascular disease, hypovolemic bird will be hypotensive, and it may be difficult to measure the pressure until some treatments are done.
- Someone must be recording the measurements and time points so that trends can be assessed.

Equipment

- Ultrasonic audio Doppler (8 Hz) with a small footprint transducer head
- Variety of inflatable cuffs, starting with the smallest neonatal size
- A hand-operated sphygmomanometer
- Recording data sheet (computer or paper!) This is often part of the vitals noted at intervals during anesthesia or surgical procedures.
- Electrode or ultrasound contact gel
- Restraint equipment (e.g. towel and restraint strap)
- Sedative or pre-anesthetic or anesthetic: Use coincides with other procedures. If part of a cardiac examination, many birds may receive IN midazolam at 2 mg/kg to allow for relaxation and a more accurate reading.
- Gauze sponges

Technical Action

1) Restrain the bird in a towel and/or restraint strap.
2) Initial measurement of BP should be done with just a sedative in effect before administration of full anesthesia. Administer a sedative of choice at this time, and wait a few minutes before taking the first measurement.
3) Depending on the size of the bird and the procedure to be done, BP can be taken using the cutaneous ulnar/wing vein and ulnar artery, which crosses over the ventral aspect of the elbow region or the metatarsal vessels of the legs. Part the feathers with a little alcohol, and using a dab of gel on the transducer, establish that an audio beat can be heard.
4) Place a cuff of appropriate size (cuff width should be 30–40% of the circumference of the limb: humerus or femur) proximally to the transducer.
5) Lock the sphygmomanometer and inflate the cuff until the heartbeat is no longer heard.
6) Very slowly release the pressure and wait for acquisition of the audio heart sound. Slowly continue the deflation until the cuff is fully deflated. Record this initial pressure where the heart sound was heard.
7) Repeat two more times. (generally, three readings are taken).
8) If during an anesthetic procedure, recovery, or critical care monitoring, repeat the process at regular intervals.
9) When completed, remove the cuff. Clean the limb with a gauze to remove contact gel/alcohol and dry the feathers.
10) If the examination is finished, release the bird slowly back into its home cage.
11) Clean and disinfect the cuff with the method recommended by the manufacturer. The transducer should also be wiped clean with alcohol, dried, and replaced in its case for protection.

Rationale/Amplification

2: Accurate BP readings cannot be taken if a bird is wrestling with the restraint, stressed (vocalizing), or in panic or pain. Using sedation (with or without an analgesic) will not interfere with collecting BP readings to assess trends.

8: Each clinic should have surgery or procedure monitoring protocols with specified intervals for collecting measurements. A staff member should be designated to do so.

Procedure

Echocardiographic imaging
Interpretation of the echocardiograph is beyond the scope of this text. This procedure will cover obtaining the views required for cardiac assessment.

Purpose

To assess the heart function, by visualization using ultrasonography

Complications

- Avian anatomy allows basically for two views of the heart, with the probe aiming craniad through the liver.
- The M-mode is not possible as the beam cannot be aimed transversely to the valves and the cardiac walls due to the position of the avian heart directly dorsal to the sternum.

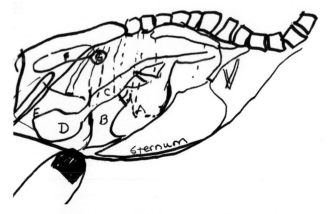

Figure 16.11 position of the probe, just under the caudal edge of the sternum, aiming up through the liver to image the heart. A: heart B: liver C: proventriculus D: ventriculus E: intestines F: kidney G: gonad.

Due to the size of the sternum and the position of the probe, obtaining views in birds less than 30 grams can be difficult. The ultrasound equipment must have a probe of 7.5 and above MHz, with a small footprint.

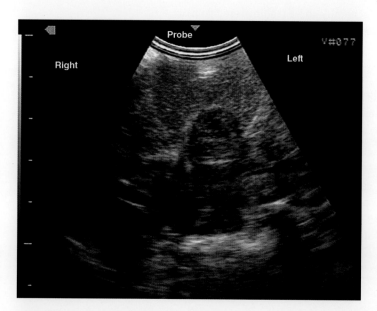

Figure 16.12 The heart will appear inverted as you are aiming through the liver. The liver and probe are at the top of the picture.

Equipment

- Ultrasound machine, transducer 7.5 MHz and above, and small footprint. The authors use one with a convex probe, but curvilinear or linear can be used. It is advantageous to have a foot pedal for instantaneous image captures.
- Recording equipment and software that allows for videos, still views, measurements (usually after the views are recorded to minimize the time the bird must be restrained), and color Doppler to assess blood flow, valve regurgitation, etc. Photographic printers are nice to send home an image with the owner, although digital images can be provided as well.
- Restraint equipment (e.g. towel, restraint strap, and even a radiographic restraint board can hold the bird in position).
- Sedatives such as midazolam to relax the bird. (2 mg/kg IN for most psittacines). This minimizes the time it takes to get the photos needed.
- Isopropyl alcohol to wet the feathers.
- Ultrasound gel for improved contact.
- Gauze sponges and towel for drying the bird after the procedure.

Technical Action

1) Restrain the bird in the towel and/or restraint strap.
2) The bird can be in dorsal recumbency, but the author prefers the bird to be held upright in a normal standing position.
3) The feathers just caudal to the sternum should be well-wetted and parted so that the skin is fully exposed. In birds with downy feathers in this area, some may need to be plucked as the feather follicles contain calcium and produce an artifact.
4) Apply a small dab of gel onto the transducer, and place the transducer somewhat under the sternum, at an angle along the interior surface of the sternum cranially.
5) The liver is used as an ultrasonic window.
6) The heart will be viewed in its long axis, and by turning the probe, two views can be obtained.
7) The image will be inverted as the beam is going through the apex of the ventricles first.

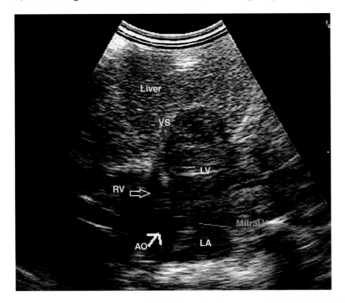

Figure 16.13 RV, right ventricle; VS, ventricular septum; LV, left ventricle; AO, aortic outflow; LA, right atrium; mitral, mitral valve (not easily seen on this still image). It is easier to see on a moving ultrasound view.

8) Photos should be taken of the entire heart, including movies to show the contraction and valve action. Rotate the transducer 90 degrees, and repeat the photos.
9) These will allow measurements of the ventricles, aortic outflow, mitral valve, atria, and overall heart size on the diastole and systole.
10) Switch to color Doppler and assess blood flow, if regurgitation is present at the valves. Record images and movies.
11) If your ultrasound machine allows for audio heart sound recordings at the same time as the video, have this feature engaged.
12) Before finishing, assess if there is free fluid around the heart or in the coelom and if other anomalies are obvious in a quick scan of the coelom.

Rationale/Amplification

2: The author prefers the bird to be at a height that the author can place the transducer comfortably under the bird aiming dorsally. If necessary, the author also places a hand on the bird's back or rump under the towel, just so that positioning the probe is done proprioceptively by the operator. A foot pedal can help take instantaneous photos when the probe is angled correctly and the view is diagnostic.

6–10: The images should be viewed after the bird has been released from restraint, and the clinician has time to make the measurements and assess the cardiac movement. Assessment of cardiac function is beyond the scope of this text.

BIBLIOGRAPHY

Casares M, Enders F, Montoya JA. Comparative electrocardiography in four species of macaws (genera Anodorhynchus and Ara). 2000. *J Vet Med A Physiol Pathol Clin Med*; 47(5): 277–281. doi: 10.1046/j.1439-0442.2000.00286.x.

Cornelia K, Krautwald-Junghanns ME. Heart disease in pet birds – diagnostic options. 2022. *Vet Clin North Am Exot Anim Pract*; 25(2): 409–433. doi: 10.1016/j.cvex.2022.01.004.

Dos Santos GJ, da Silva JP, Hippólito AG, Ferro BS, Oliveira ELR, Okamoto PTCG, Lourenço MLG, de Vasconcelos Machado VM, Rahal SC, Teixeira CR, Melchert A. Computed tomographic and radiographic morphometric study of cardiac and coelomic dimensions in captive blue-fronted Amazon parrots (*Amazona aestiva*, Linnaeus, 1758) with varying body condition scores. 2020. *Anat Histol Embryol*; 49(2): 299–306. doi: 10.1111/ahe.12528.

Johnson-Delaney CA. Practical avian cardiology. 2006. *Exotic DVM*; 8(3): 78–85.

Straub J, Pees M, Krautwald-Junghanns ME. Measurement of the cardiac silhouette in psittacines. 2002. *J Am Vet Med Assoc*; 221(1): 76–79. doi: 10.2460/javma.2002.221.76.

Strunk A, Wilson GH. Avian cardiology. 2003. *Vet Clin North Am Exot Anim Pract*; 6(1): 1–28.

17

Hemostasis

Purpose

To stop hemorrhage from wounds.

A hematoma is a site of hemorrhage under the skin or within an organ or body cavity. It is also known as a bruise. As a bruise resolves, it becomes fibrotic. It may cause contraction of the affective tissues. Generally, they will resolve without treatment.

- When an injury that causes a hematoma happens and can be treated immediately (such as leakage following a catheter removal or blood draw), direct manual digital pressure may prevent a large hematoma from occurring or spreading. The use of a cold pack may also speed up the clotting time and decrease the bleeding by cooling/contraction of the blood vessel. Any injured bird should have a full workup as soon as bleeding has been controlled and the bird is stabilized and no longer in shock. Usually, no further treatment is needed.

Equipment

- Restraint supplies such as towels
- Cotton and gauze
- Gentle skin cleansing solution such as 2% chlorhexidine
- Bandage materials: tape, gauze roll, and self-stick wrap (Vetrap-type)
- Hemostatic sponges

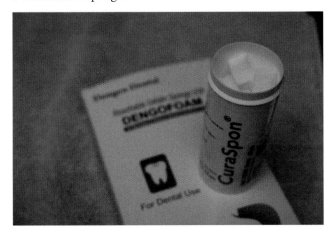

Figure 17.1 Hemostatic sponges: many commercial brands are available. Small sizes can be obtained through dental suppliers. Source: Curaspon.

Manual of Clinical Procedures in Pet Birds, First Edition. Cathy A. Johnson-Delaney and Tracy Bennett.
© 2025 John Wiley & Sons, Inc. Published 2025 by John Wiley & Sons, Inc.
Companion website: www.wiley.com/go/johnson-delaney/manual

Technical Action

1) Wounds in birds are similar to those in other animals.
2) The first step is to stop the bleeding and ascertain the seriousness of the wound.
3) If the wound is deep, it may require suturing and the bird should be prepped for surgery, with a temporary bandage or manual pressure in place during the preparation.
4) If the bleeding can be controlled manually and the wound determined to be one that can be treated just with bandaging, then once the bleeding has stopped, it can be cleansed with the surgical solution, gently dried with a cotton or gauze, and then bandaged with a wet–dry bandage.
5) Hemostatic sponges can be applied directly to the wound to stop bleeding and can be incorporated in the dressing.

Rationale/Amplification

Parenteral antibiotics, analgesics, and potentially NSAIDs are usually needed when there is a bleeding wound, as many times, there are deep punctures that are difficult to see (like from a dog or cat).
The type of dressing and duration of the bandaging is determined by the wound severity.
Discuss the options for wound healing with the owner and the likelihood that there will be discoloration in the area just like in other animals. Owners may be alarmed by the greenish look to the skin in the area post-hemorrhage.
The bird should be monitored to make sure bleeding does not resume. The bird may need some sort of a collar to prevent it from chewing the bandage.

BLOOD FEATHERS

Procedure

Bleeding blood feathers

Equipment

- Hemostats and sterile hemostats
- Needle-nosed pliers
- Restraint supplies such as a towel.
- Cotton for manual bleeding control.
- A growing feather has a blood vessel within it.
- Damage to a blood feather can cause copious bleeding.
- While hemostatic agents applied may stop the bleeding in the short term, this is not advised as it will bleed again.
- Bleeding blood feathers should be extracted. Wing and tail feathers are the most commonly presented because of damage causing the bleeding.

Technical Action

1) Restrain the bird. Sedation and/or anesthesia may be needed if the bird is severely stressed.
2) The wing (or tail) must be securely braced to protect it from trauma during the extraction if the feather is on the wing or tail. Smaller feathers on the body can also bleed and may need to be removed similarly to how a feather is plucked.

3) For most birds, hemostats are used. Large birds may require larger tools such as needle-nosed pliers.
4) Grasp the calamus of the bleeding feather, close to the skin.

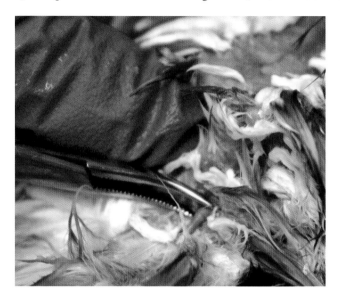

Figure 17.2   Use hemostats to grasp the base of the bleeding feather close to the skin.

5) Firmly and steadily, without twisting the feather, apply traction in the direction of the natural feather growth and pull the feather and its base from the follicle.

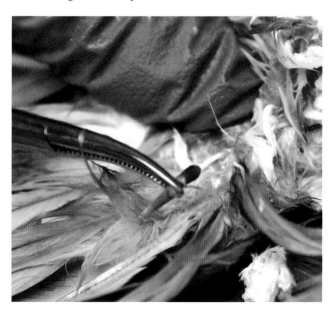

Figure 17.3   Firmly and steadily pull the feather in the direction of its growth.

6) Manual pressure with a bit of cotton is all that is usually necessary to stop any residual bleeding.

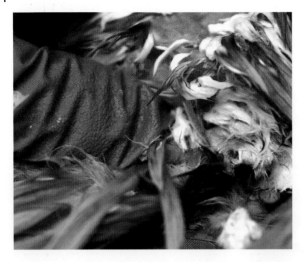

Figure 17.4   Gentle digital pressure usually with cotton or gauze will stop any residual bleeding.

7) If the feather is split or shredded within the base of the calamus, it may be necessary to use sterile hemostats, inserted into the shaft, and grasp the wall to extract it.

Rationale/Amplification

Feathers should be extracted with traction in the direction of the feather growth so as not to damage the periosteum and follicles.
Flight feathers are attached to the bone by the periosteum.
Occasionally, an open follicle is very large, and a drop of tissue glue can be used to close it. Be aware that it could be a chewing point for the bird. Most follicle openings do not need to be surgically closed.
Remind the owner that the bird's flight and balance may be affected by the removal of the feather and that they should use caution when the bird is out of its cage.
It is not recommended that owners extract blood feathers at home: it may result in further feather damage and/or fractures.

TOENAILS

Procedure

Bleeding toenail hemostasis

Purpose

Most pet birds require toenail trimming periodically as the nails are not worn down like they are in the wild.

Some birds have white nails, and many larger psittacines have pigmented (gray to black) nails where the quick cannot be directly visualized.

Clipping should be done by someone knowledgeable so that the quick is not penetrated.

Equipment

● Appropriately sized toenail clippers. There are several commercial ones available for various animals that may work. Usually personal preference, but best to avoid clippers that squeeze or compress the nail as that causes discomfort. Gauze, cotton. Hemostatic agents: silver nitrate sticks, powder, liquid, hemostatic sponges. There are cautery devices available, but these can cause burns and pain and the authors do not recommend their usage. Bandage supplies for longer direct pressure on a bleeding nail if a few minutes does not seem adequate.

Technical Action

1) Restrain the bird so that the bleeding nail can be isolated and worked with.
2) While holding the digit and bleeding nail, wipe the nail with a gauze sponge, and if the blood has spread to many toes and the foot, the foot will need to be cleaned.

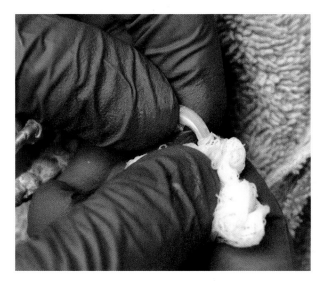

Figure 17.5 Cleanse the nail to determine the volume of hemorrhage.

3) Gently squeeze the bleeding toe slightly. This digital pressure may slow or stop the bleeding.
4) To the tip of the nail that is bleeding, hemostatic powder, solution, or a sponge can be applied along with digital pressure. Usually, bleeding will stop within a few minutes.

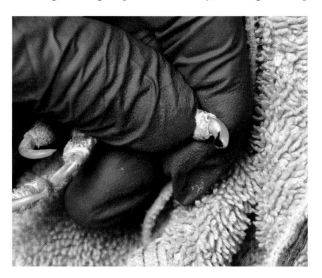

Figure 17.6 Hold the nail to determine extent of damage and bleeding.

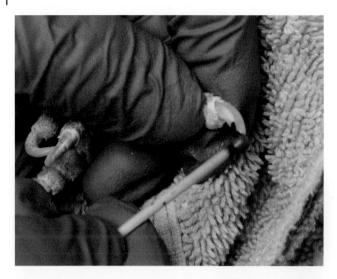

Figure 17.7   Use of a silver nitrate stick. Note: this can be irritating. It will cause dark brown stains on hands, towels, etc.

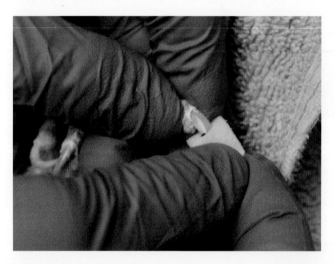

Figure 17.8   Use of a hemostatic sponge.

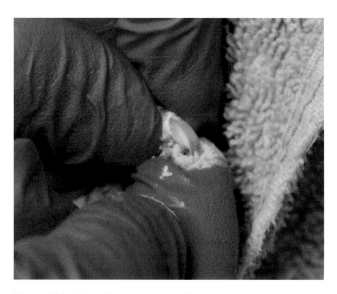

Figure 17.9   Use of hemostatic powder.

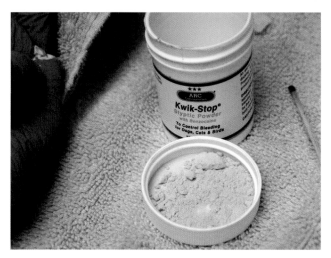

Figure 17.10   Commonly used hemostatic agents, although many commercial types can be used.

5) If seepage or very slight bleeding continues, a bandage may be applied that keeps pressure on the tip of the quick that is bleeding.

Rationale/Amplification

Some use battery-operated portable cautery units to cauterize the tip. This is quick; however, it does cause some pain. The owner may also be unhappy with the smell (cooking meat) that occurs at the cautery.

A bandage for a bleeding toenail usually only needs to stay on for 15–30 minutes. The bandage needs to stay on long enough for clotting to have occurred. A bird that immediately pulls a bandage off may sometimes pull the newly formed clot off, and bleeding starts again.

The amount of blood lost from a toenail is minor; however, birds seem to spread it all over a perch and cage, making it look far worse than it is.

BIBLIOGRAPHY

Bowles HL, Odberg E, Harrison GJ, Kottwitz JJ. Surgical resolution of soft tissue disorders. In: Harrison GJ, Lightfoot TL (eds). *Clinical Avian Medicine Volume II*. 2006. Spix Publishing, Inc., Palm Beach, FL. pp 775–829.

Harrison GJ, Woerpel RW, Rosskopf WJ Jr, Karpinski LG. Symptomatic therapy and emergency medicine. In: *Clinical Avian Medicine and Surgery Including Aviculture*. 1986. WB Saunders Co., Philadelphia, PA. pp 362–375.

18

Transfusions

Purpose

A transfusion is indicated if a bird's PCV is less than 20% or if there has been hemorrhage of more than 3 mL/100 grams of body weight. Other indications are severe emaciation, kidney/liver disease with anemia, and/or coagulopathy.

It is preferable to have a donor bird of the same species available; however, studies have shown that one trans-avian species transfusion can provide some benefit. The closer the donor species is to the recipient, the more the erythrocyte lifespan is prolonged. If a second transfusion is needed, cross-matching should be done.

Equipment

- Donor bird(s)
- Sedatives and anesthetics
- Small blood transfusion bags with a filter for infusion. Anticoagulants should be citrate. If the volume to be used is small, rather than using a transfusion bag and filter, citrate should be added to the syringe of blood at a 5:1 ratio. Gentle rocking of the syringe with the fresh blood and citrate will thoroughly mix it.
- Appropriate catheter and placement such as an IO catheter in the recipient prior to removal of the blood from the donor should be performed.

Technical Action

1) The donor bird is sedated and/or anesthetized for the blood draw. This bird should be kept warm until recovered.
2) The recipient bird is usually sedated and/or anesthetized for IO or IV catheter placement.
3) The fresh blood with citrate should be injected slowly preferably through a catheter as a bolus of 5 mL/100 grams body weight.
4) The bird should be monitored as it recovers, usually in a warm incubator-type setting.

Rationale/Amplification

The volume of blood needed should be based on 5 mL/100 grams body weight.
Supplemental injections of vitamin B complex, iron, and vitamin K may also be administered.
If a second bolus is needed, it is usually administered at least 24 hours later to avoid circulatory distress.

Manual of Clinical Procedures in Pet Birds, First Edition. Cathy A. Johnson-Delaney and Tracy Bennett.
© 2025 John Wiley & Sons, Inc. Published 2025 by John Wiley & Sons, Inc.
Companion website: www.wiley.com/go/johnson-delaney/manual

Additional Considerations and Treatments

1) Alternative fluids if blood transfusion is unavailable
2) Oxyglobin (hemoglobin glutamer-200-bovine) at 30 mL/kg IV once
3) Hetastarch: 10–15 mL/kg IV q 8 h up to four treatments
4) Additional treatment for anemia:
5) Erythropoietin at 100 IU/kg SC 3 X a week until PCV has recovered.

BIBLIOGRAPHY

Harrison GJ, Lightfoot TL, Flinchum GB. Emergency and critical care. In: Harrison GJ, Lightfoot TL (eds). *Clinical Avian Medicine Volume I.* 2006. Spix Publishing, Inc., Palm Beach, FL. pp 213–231.

Wöst E, Lierz M. The thin bird. In: Chitty J, Monks D (eds). *BSAVA Manual of Avian Practice. A Foundation Manual.* 2018. British Small Animal Veterinary Association, Quedgeley, UK. pp 377–388.

19

Air Sac Cannulation and Oxygen Supplementation

Purpose

Severe dyspnea due to obstruction in the trachea

An alternative method to deliver additional oxygen or inhalant anesthesia.

Complications

The body cavity or air sacs filled with a fluid or a mass preventing access to the air sacs.

This is not used for air sacculitis, or respiratory disease caudal to the syrinx, or non-respiratory dyspnea (such as neoplasia or organomegaly that is compressing the air sacs).

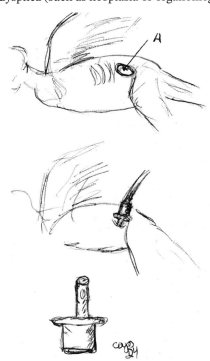

Figure 19.1 The bird is on the right lateral side. A. Paralumbar area to access the abdomen and air sac. The second drawing shows the air sac cannula inserted, and the bottom picture is an example of a short air sac cannula. The tube should be sterile, and the adapter fits a hose for delivery of oxygen. A. Paralumbar area for the incision.

Manual of Clinical Procedures in Pet Birds, First Edition. Cathy A. Johnson-Delaney and Tracy Bennett.
© 2025 John Wiley & Sons, Inc. Published 2025 by John Wiley & Sons, Inc.
Companion website: www.wiley.com/go/johnson-delaney/manual

Equipment

- Oxygen delivery system to attach or cover the air sac cannula
- Cannula: this can be fashioned from an endotracheal tube of a size larger than the bird's trachea: cut the tube so that it is long enough to access the air sac, usually about 2 cm, but depends on the size of the bird. The advantage of this is that the connection end of the tube will fit readily to an oxygen or anesthetic delivery system. Alternatively, in emergencies, a cut red rubber tube or urinary catheter can be used. The tube must be long enough to extend beyond the bird's body to attach to the oxygen/anesthesia machine adapters with hoses. Red rubber catheters can also be modified for this. Commercial avian air sac cannulas are available and come with a retention disc attached for ease of attachment to the skin.
- Suture or glue or tape
- # 15 scalpel blade
- Hemostatic forceps
- Isopropyl alcohol and gauze sponges
- Skin antiseptic/surgery prep solution
- Lidocaine 2% with a syringe and needle (preferably 25–27 ga, 0.5-mL syringe)
- Anesthesia machine if gas anesthesia is to be connected to the cannula, with appropriate adapters, tubes, and hoses.
- Antibiotic cream

Technical Action

1) *Note*: this is usually an emergency procedure; although radiographs and/or ultrasonography can aid in assessment of the abdomen, usually the cannula is placed to allow respiration, and then other diagnostics are done. The site of placement is similar to that for lateral laparoscopy.
2) Place the bird in right lateral recumbency.
3) Wet the skin and feathers over the area of the left caudal air sac (paralumbar area, just caudal to the eighth or last rib) using alcohol.
4) Infiltrate the skin at the insertion point with 0.05–0.1 mL lidocaine (depends on the size of the bird).
5) Cleanse skin with a surgical prep solution.
6) Make a stab incision at the site.
7) Using the hemostats, push through the abdominal wall and into the air sac.
8) Insert the cannula.
9) Manipulate it so that it is not up against an organ. You should immediately note the change in respiration and be able to see moisture vapor in the tube. A down feather can be used to test for air movement (breathing).
10) When the tube is properly placed, it can be sutured to the skin incision using either the finger trap method or butterfly tape and suture it around the tube. If a commercial cannula with a retention disc is used, it can be sutured to the skin. Additionally, you can add a drop of glue at the site to help hold the tube in place.
11) Put a small amount of antibiotic cream on the skin around the tube.
12) As the bird moves and respiration improves, and once the bird is standing, adjustments in the placement of the tube may be needed. It should be monitored.
13) The tube may remain in place for several days.

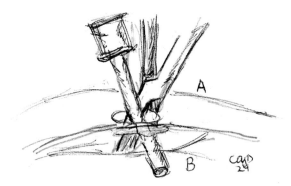

Figure 19.2 The cannula is inserted through the incision in the skin and body wall and into the air sac using hemostats. The cannula can be of varying lengths but should have a standard adapter attached that can fit with oxygen or an anesthesia machine. A: Skin B. Air sac.

Rationale/Amplification

\# The cannula provides an alternate airway.

\# It can be replaced as needed while the primary airway obstruction is resolved.

\# Gas anesthesia can be administered through the cannula the same way it is managed through an endotracheal tube.

\# When tracheal respiration is restored, the cannula can be removed.

\# The abdomen/skin may be sutured or the skin glued. Some may just be allowed to close spontaneously.

BIBLIOGRAPHY

Harrison GJ, Lightfoot TL, Flinchum GB. Emergency and critical care. In: Harrison GJ, Lightfoot TL (eds). *Clinical Avian Medicine Volume I*. 2006. Spix Publishing, Inc., Palm Beach, FL. pp 213–231.

Quesenberry KE, Hillyer EV. Supportive care and emergency therapy. In: Ritchie BW, Harrison GJ, Harrison LR (eds). *Avian Medicine: Principles and Applications*. 1994. Wingers Publishing, Inc., Lake Worth, FL. pp 352–416.

20

CPR (Cardiopulmonary Resuscitation)

Cardiopulmonary resuscitation (CPR) in birds follows the same guidelines as used in mammals. However, due to the presence of the keel (sternum), direct palpation and massage of the heart is not possible. Prognosis is found to be poor, and owners need to be informed that this is a critical condition. Some texts describe cardiopulmonary resuscitation (CPR) as CPCR, which is cardiopulmonary cerebral resuscitation.

CPR attempts to maintain oxygenation and perfusion of the brain and vital organs while attempting to restore spontaneous respiration and circulation. The underlying events or disease processes that result in cardiopulmonary arrest (CPA) include cardiac disease, hypovolemia (including trauma hemorrhage), renal disease, electrolyte imbalances, metabolic disorders (liver and kidney), systemic inflammation, respiratory compromise, and sedation/anesthesia. The cause(s) must be considered as it influences the probability of success. CPCR has the best chance of success following acute fluid or blood loss or if it occurs during anesthesia.

The only contraindication to performing CPCR is if there is a do-not-resuscitate (DNR) directive from the owner. Many anesthesia consent forms include this caveat for the owner to be aware of the potential and what they wish the clinician to do during a CPA event.

If the CPA occurs outside of the hospital, the faster the bird is presented to the hospital, the more the success rate is affected. In mammals, it is thought that if CPR is started within 5 minutes, there may be a chance for recovery. However, in birds, that time may be shorter as their metabolic needs are higher. At present, there has been little scientific evidence for the optimal time interval for resuscitation.

If the CPA occurs in the hospital, immediate intervention can occur. In a published study, the survival rate was still poor and contributed to the difficulty delivering good chest/thorax compressions, accessing the circulation, performing defibrillation, and other anatomic/physiologic attributes. While birds may be resuscitated in the short term, long-term prognosis is poor.

A "crash cart" specifically for avian patients should be maintained and placed in a central, easy-to-access location in the hospital. This cart should be enclosed so that it remains sealed between uses. This stops the removal of critical supplies – it should have a supply list and checklist for replenishment that must be initialed by the individual who re-stocks it. The cart is then sealed such that it will be obvious if that seal is broken. There should also be a quick chart of the drugs to be used inside the cart – dosages by weight Table 20.1.

Manual of Clinical Procedures in Pet Birds, First Edition. Cathy A. Johnson-Delaney and Tracy Bennett.
© 2025 John Wiley & Sons, Inc. Published 2025 by John Wiley & Sons, Inc.
Companion website: www.wiley.com/go/johnson-delaney/manual

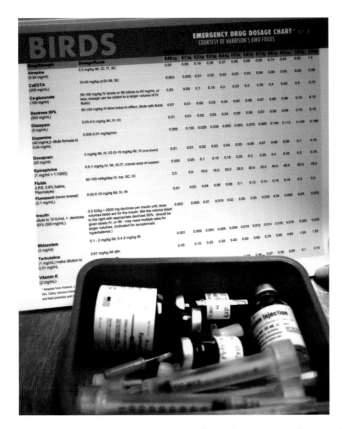

Figure 20.1 Emergency drug kit containing dosage chart, drugs, and syringes.

Anesthesia-related CPA may have the best chance of resuscitation, mainly because an airway will already be established (intubation) and usually venous access is established (either IV or IO catheter). Oxygen is immediately available. Birds may have more profound respiratory depression with many inhalant anesthetic agents and even sedatives/opioids, although careful consideration of dosing in light of more pharmacologic research studies being done in various species can help alleviate much of the risk. Hypotension and arrhythmias likely precede many of the arrests and can be closely monitored now during anesthesia. There are a number of ECG and blood pressure systems available that are suitable for avian heart rates (see Chapter 10). Maintaining the bird's body temperature is also critical for maintaining circulation and metabolism.

Arrhythmias, hypotension (circulatory shock), and bradycardia should be addressed immediately before respiratory or cardiac arrest occurs. These can be mediated by different drugs (atropine, glycopyrrolate, vasopressors, epinephrine, doxapram, etc.) along with adjusting the fluid therapy and inhalant anesthetic levels, which can prevent CPA.

Purpose

To provide CPR immediately after the CPA is determined.

Table 20.1 Emergency avian drugs.

Exotic animal drug dosage chart – courtesy of Harrison's bird foods

BIRDS

Dose volume (in bold) is listed for a low dose if the range is given

Drug/Strength	Dosage/Route	0.05 kg	0.1 kg	0.2 kg	0.3 kg	0.4 kg	0.5 kg	0.6 kg	0.7 kg	0.8 kg	0.9 kg	1.0 kg	1.5 kg
Aminophylline (25 mg/mL)	**4 mg/kg PO, IM q12h; 10 mg/kg** IVq3h	0.01	0.02	0.03	0.05	0.06	0.08	0.1	0.11	0.13	0.14	0.16	0.24
Atropine (0.54 mg/mL)	0.5 mg/kg IM, IO, IT, SC	0.05	0.09	0.19	0.28	0.37	0.46	0.56	0.65	0.74	0.83	0.93	1.4
CaEDTA (200 mg/mL)	10–40 mg/kg q12h IM, SC	0.003	0.005	0.01	0.02	0.02	0.03	0.03	0.04	0.04	0.05	0.05	0.08
Ca-gluconate (100 mg/mL)	50–100 mg/kg IV slowly or IM (dilute to 50 mg/mL or less; the dosage can be added to a larger volume of IV fluids)	0.03	0.05	0.1	0.15	0.2	0.25	0.3	0.35	0.4	0.45	0.5	0.75
Dexamethasone (NaSP) (4 mg/mL)	2–4 mg/kg IV, IM (comment: Use cautiously, an immunosuppressive effect)	0.03	0.05	0.1	0.15	0.2	0.25	0.3	0.35	0.4	0.45	0.5	0.75
Dextrose 50% (500 mg/mL)	50–100 mg/kg IV slow bolus to effect, dilute with fluids	0.01	0.01	0.02	0.03	0.04	0.05	0.06	0.07	0.08	0.09	0.10	0.15
Diazepam (5 mg/mL)	**0.5–1.0 mg/kg** IM, IV, IO	0.01	0.01	0.02	0.03	0.04	0.05	0.06	0.07	0.08	0.09	0.10	0.15
Dopamine (40 mg/mL): dilute formula to 0.04 mg/mL)	0.005–0.01 mg/kg/min	0.006	0.130	0.025	0.038	0.050	0.063	0.075	0.088	0.100	0.113	0.125	0.188
Doxapram (20 mg/mL)	2 mg/kg IM, IV, IO	0.01	0.01	0.02	0.03	0.04	0.05	0.06	0.07	0.08	0.09	0.1	0.15
Epinephrine (1 mg/ mL = 1:1000)	**0.5–1 mg/kg** IV, IM, IO, IT, cranial area of the coelom	0.025	0.05	0.1	0.15	0.19	0.25	0.3	0.35	0.4	0.45	0.5	0.75
Fluids (LRS, 0.9% saline)	50–100 mL/kg/day IV, ice, SC, and IO	2.5	5.0	10.0	15.0	20.0	25.0	30.0	35.0	40.0	45.0	50.0	75.0
Flumazenil (benzo reversal) (0.1 mg/mL)	**0.02**–0.10 mg/kg IM, IV, and IN	0.01	0.02	0.04	0.06	0.08	0.1	0.12	0.14	0.16	0.18	0.2	0.3

Drug												
Insulin dilute to 10 IU/ mL + dextrose 50% (500 mg/mL) 0.5 IU/kg + 2000 mg dextrose per insulin unit; dose volumes listed are for the insulin. Mix the volume listed to the right with appropriate dextrose 50%: should be given slowly IV, or IM – may need multiple sites for larger volumes.	0.003	0.005	0.01	0.015	0.02	0.25	0.03	0.035	0.04	0.045	0.05	0.075
Midazolam (5 mg/ml) 0.1–2 mg/kg IM; 0.4–2 mg/kg IN	0.001	0.002	0.004	0.006	0.008	0.010	0.012	0.014	0.016	0.018	0.020	0.030
Terbutaline (1 mg/mL) make dilution to **0.01 mg/ mL** 0.01 mg/kg IM q6h	0.05	0.10	0.20	0.30	0.40	0.50	0.60	0.70	0.80	0.90	1.00	1.50
Vitamin K (2 mg/mL) **0.2**–2.2 mg/kg IM Q4–8 h until stable then once Q24H	0.005	0.01	0.02	0.03	0.04	0.05	0.06	0.07	0.08	0.09	0.1	0.15

Reference Chart for Exotic Animals. Exotic DVM 5.5 pp 23–24, 2003. Reviewed and Updated by Drs. Cathy Johnson-Delaney and Vanessa Rolfe, 2023. This chart is provided as a courtesy by HBD International, Inc. (HBD). All users assume sole responsibility for its proper use in accordance with medical regulations and best practices and hold HBD harmless for any liability that may relate to its use.
Source: Adapted from Kottwitz J, Kelleher S: Emergency Drugs.

Complications

- Length of time between CPA and intervention with CPR – the longer the interval, the less likely there will be success.
- Unknown underlying medical conditions.
- Lack of immediate intravenous access and airway access.
- Lack of monitoring such as ECG and blood pressure that allow the clinician to adjust therapies.
- No well-stocked crash cart and lack of staff trained to deal with CPA.

Equipment

- Oxygen, masks, endotracheal tubes, and attachment hoses
- ECG monitor
- Doppler audio monitor, sphygmomanometer, appropriate sizes of cuffs; electronic blood pressure monitor
- Pulse oximeter, side-stream capnographic probe.
- Assortment of avian-sized intravenous catheters; needles appropriate for IO catheters; catheter plug
- Assortment of needles and syringes
- Fluids – saline, D5W, LRS, etc.
- Drugs: see Table 20.1
- Tape (to secure catheter, mask, etc.)
- Stethoscopes
- Anesthesia machine, ventilator, and syringe pump (these may be in the surgery already)
- Incubator/critical care caging module, capable of receiving oxygen
- Patient warming system. Note: fluid volumes appropriate for the patient can be drawn up and warmed using the patient system.

Technical Action

1) If on inhalant anesthetics or receiving intravenous anesthetics – stop administration immediately.
2) Begin thoracic compressions. These are usually done one-handed in the pet bird, with the thumb and forefinger doing the compressions dorso/ventro, approximately as much as normal excursion, but as fast as possible (at least 120 compressions/min).

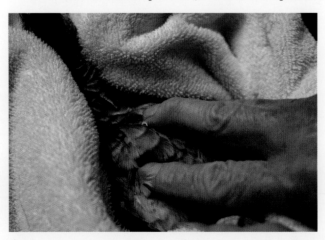

Figure 20.2 Place two fingers on either side of the sternum, and gently start rapid compressions.

3) Place a large mask over the bird's head and start the oxygen, while readying to intubate, if not already intubated. While doing thoracic compression, another team member should intubate the bird and secure the tube.

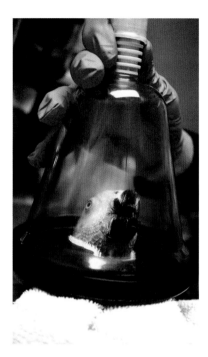

Figure 20.3 While preparing to intubate, start oxygen therapy using a large mask fitted entirely over the head. When intubated, this same mask can be used to provide oxygen. Alternatively, an Ambu bag can be used to give gentle pumps of air or oxygen either with or without an endotracheal tube in place. Be careful not to over-ventilate – tiny puffs only.

4) Hold an oxygen mask over the tube ("flow-by") so that with thoracic compression, oxygen is being respirated. Every 15–30 seconds, do a positive pressure "sigh" with the oxygen attached to the tube, inflating the thorax to an approximately normal position. The person doing the compressions stops for this quick "breath" and resumes immediately after.

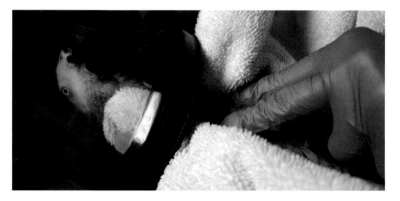

5) If not already attached to cardiac and respiratory monitors, a team member should be hooking the bird up. Preferably, the person doing the thoracic compressions is also monitoring with a stethoscope for heartbeat.
   a) ECG leads attach to the skin of the axillae and thigh patagiums.
   b) Leads can be attached using hypodermic needles, paper clips, gel-soaked gauzes, self-adhesive patches, or loops (depending on the monitoring equipment). A dab of electrode gel will improve contact.
6) Another team member should establish vascular access, and once established, bolus fluids can be administered. Generally, the volume can be based on 25 mL/kg/hour but adjusted per blood pressure. Ideally, fluids should be warmed to close to body temperature.
7) Another team member should take the blood pressure.
   a) The Doppler probe is used on the proximal ulna or the medial tibiotarsus.
   b) Cuff width should be 30–40% of the circumference of the limb: humerus or femur.
   c) Monitors trends rather than absolute systolic pressure.
8) Watch the ECG for signs of a heartbeat.
9) If no heartbeat after 30 seconds, administer epinephrine and doxapram and continue chest compressions.
10) Repeated or additional drugs can be administered after 1–2 minutes if no effect.
11) Discontinue compressions every minute to assess for return to spontaneous circulation (ECG, Doppler, and auscultation).
12) Generally, if spontaneous sinus rhythm and respiration have not been established within 5–7 minutes of the above, and at least two doses of many of the drugs, resuscitation is deemed unsuccessful.
13) If spontaneous sinus rhythm and respirations resume, discontinue chest compressions, and keep oxygen support going. Continue to monitor the bird until it is conscious and standing. This usually means placement in a metabolic cage or incubator, maintaining electronic monitoring until ambulatory, adjusting fluid therapy, and monitoring blood pressure for potentially hours after the CPA event. With recovery, additional diagnostics may be needed including blood drawn for electrolyte and metabolite levels and additional imaging. Ideally, a nurse should be assigned to monitor the bird continuously following such an event until the bird is sufficiently recovered to be discharged from the hospital.

Rationale/Amplification

1–10 effectively are occurring simultaneously. Staff members must be trained for their roles, and this procedure is practiced in mock situations.

11. This timing can be arbitrary – but called by the veterinarian.

12. During recovery and intensive care, the bird's condition should be evaluated as to "why" it occurred, and further investigation of underlying causes takes place.

BIBLIOGRAPHY

Johnson-Delaney CA, Rolfe V. Birds. In: Johnson-Delaney CA, Rolfe V (eds). *Exotic Animal Drug Dosage Chart*. 2023. Harrison's Bird Diets, Brentwood, TN.

Kabakchiev C, Beaufrere H. CPR and euthanasia. In: Graham JE, Doss GA, Beaufrere H (eds). *Exotic Animal Emergency and Critical Care Medicine*. 2021. Wiley Blackwell, Hoboken, NJ. Chapter 32, electronic edition, no page numbers visible.

21

Fluid Therapy

Purpose

- Rehydration for any dehydrated bird.
- Supplying fluids during surgery to maintain normal perfusion.

Equipment

- Fluids: Plasma-lyte, Normasol-R, or 0.9% sodium chloride are preferred.
- Regular lactated ringers can be used.
- Hypertonic saline.
- Catheters for intravenous, intraosseous, or subcutaneous administration.
- Spinal needles, hypodermic needles, and various gauges.
- Syringe infusion pump.
- Various syringes, feeding tubes, or crop needles to administer oral fluids.
- Oral speculums, various sizes and types.
- Rehydration commercial formulations.

Technical Action

Fluids can be delivered orally, subcutaneously, intravenously, or intraosseously. Fluids should be warmed to avian body temperature for administration.

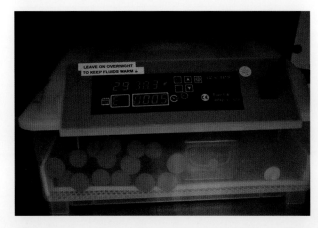

Figure 21.1 Incubator utilized to keep fluids warmed for immediate use.

Manual of Clinical Procedures in Pet Birds, First Edition. Cathy A. Johnson-Delaney and Tracy Bennett.
© 2025 John Wiley & Sons, Inc. Published 2025 by John Wiley & Sons, Inc.
Companion website: www.wiley.com/go/johnson-delaney/manual

ORAL FLUIDS

Crop needles or tubes are easy to use to administer a calculated volume of the rehydration solution.

Crop needle/stainless steel with a ball on the tip:

Example of sizes: Budgerigar: 18 ga

Cockatiel/conures: 16 ga

Amazons, grays, and small cockatoos: 10–12 ga

Macaws and larger cockatoos: 14 ga or more and longer at 16–20 cm

1) Calculation of the amount of the fluid: 2–3% of an adult bird's body weight per oral feeding is the volume safe to use. Compare this to the volume required to correct the hydration and determine the frequency needed over a 24-hour period.
2) Restrain the bird manually.
3) Insert the crop needle into the mouth from the bird's left commissure.

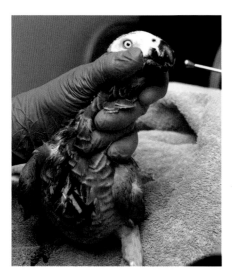

Figure 21.2 Showing the approach to insertion of the feeding needle.

4) Some will clamp down hard: if this happens, try rotating it slightly while gently continuing to insert it. Usually, you are able to then pass it across the tongue and down into the crop.
5) Confirm the tip is in the crop: palpate the tip using the thumb or finger against the crop wall. You can also move it against the crop wall and skin. Note: if it is in the trachea, generally the bird will be fighting and gasping at this point, but if not, you would not be able to palpate the tip.
6) Inject a small amount of the fluid and watch the bird's reaction. If it ignores the process, then you are definitely in the crop, not the trachea.

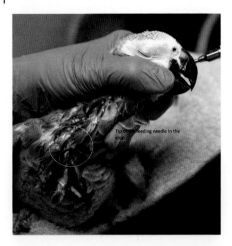

Tip of the feeding needle in the crop

Figure 21.3 The feeding needle is inserted into the crop.

7) Proceed to inject the fluids into the crop, and remove the needle as soon as all are delivered.
8) If you are using a red rubber, flexible-type feeding tube, you may need an oral speculum to prevent the bird from clamping down on the tube.

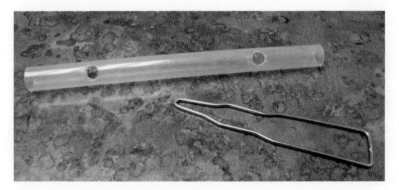

Figure 21.4 Two different types of speculums for use with birds to aid in passage of feeding tube.

9) You can confirm the tip is in the crop the same way as for a rigid needle.
10) Once the fluids are delivered, crimp the tube to withdraw it (similarly to what is done during gavage feeding to prevent the fluid from leaking out during the withdrawing process).
11) If the fluid regurgitates back into the pharynx, the crop is likely overfilled. Immediately, place the bird in its cage or even an oxygenated cage to allow it to regurgitate the fluid and swallow the excess without aspiration.

SUBCUTANEOUS

1) The preferred location for SC fluid administration in psittacines is the inguinal area, into the flap of skin between the abdomen and the medial upper femur.

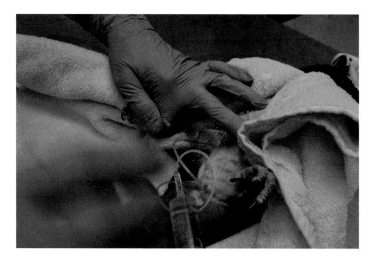

Figure 21.5   Needle placed to administer subcutaneous fluids in the inguinal web.

2) This area allows for a large volume to be injected. (up to 20 mL/kg).
3) An alternate area is the subscapular region.
4) Higher doses of fluids may lead to edema, particularly if circulation is poor.

INTRAVENOUS

1) Preferred route during hypovolemic shock or in collapsed patients.
2) The jugular, basilic, and medial metatarsal veins are most commonly used.
3) If possible, a catheter is placed, which will allow additional boluses or continuous fluid therapy.
4) A small (24–26 gauge) over-the-needle nonstick-coated catheter is guided into the vein. It is then butterflied with a tape and secured with acrylic glue or sutures to the skin.

Figure 21.6 A   This is placement of an IV catheter in a chicken, but demonstrating the tarsal positioning.

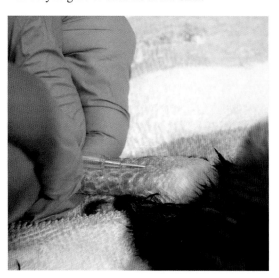

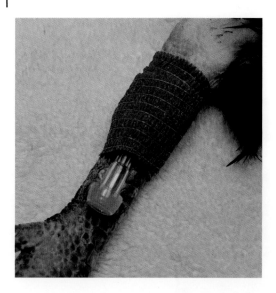

Figure 21.6 B   Shows the catheter secured with cap.

5) If the basilic vein is catheterized, the wing needs to be wrapped in a figure-of-eight bandage to prevent movement.
6) If a jugular catheter is placed, the neck needs to be wrapped lightly in cotton padding and self-adherent bandages to keep the catheter from kinking with neck movement.
7) Fluids are normally administered by slow bolus.
8) Problems associated with the use of IV fluid administration include that the bird may need to be sedated or anesthetized to have a catheter placed, as manual restraint may not be adequate. Also, the catheter, injection cap, and any tubing must be protected from the bird chewing them.
9) With a catheter in place, the bird can be connected to fluids delivered by a syringe pump. However, the tubing must be secured and protected from the bird being able to chew it. Plastic power-line type line protectors as used for dogs can be used to protect the fluid line.
10) Hematoma formation at the site of venipuncture is common, particularly if the basilic vein is used.
11) Parrots tend to work on the bandages and remove catheters as they recover.

INTRAOSSEOUS

1) The placement of an interosseous catheter allows for similar vascular access, as does the intravenous route. It is sometimes faster to place one and may cause less vascular damage than an intravenous catheter.
2) Do not use a pneumatized bone.
3) This is considered a painful procedure, so the bird should receive analgesics (parenteral and local) and/or be anesthetized for the procedure. The bird is placed in dorsal recumbency with the leg or wing to be used extended.
4) The skin over the insertion point should be surgically prepped and infiltrated with lidocaine.

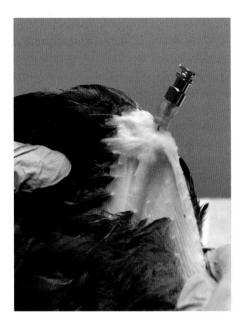

Figure 21.7   Placement in the ulna. The tibiotarsus or the ulna are the two most commonly used sites.

5) Needles to be used:
   a) Specialized bone needles, spinal needles of appropriate length, or standard syringe needle, which should be filled with fluid during insertion to prevent boney material and marrow from clogging it.
   b) <100 grams body weight: 27–30-gauge standard needle.
   c) <200 grams body weight: 23-gauge, 20-mm needle.
   d) 200–700 grams body weight: 21-gauge, 25-mm needle.
   e) >700 grams body weight: 18-gauge, 38-mm needle.
6) **For tibiotarsal placement**: Grasp the tibiotarsus in one hand and use the thumb and index finger to locate the tibiotarsal bone.

Figure 21.8   Interosseous catheter placement in the proximal tibiotarsus. A: Femur. B: Cnemial crest. C: Fibula. D: Tibiotarsus.

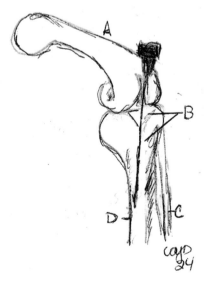

7) The needle is inserted into the cnemial crest through the insertion of the patellar tendon, which is aligned with the diaphysis. Use gentle pressure on the needle as you rotate it slightly as you insert it. Advance the needle to approximately one-third to one-half of the length of the bone.

8) Make a tape "butterfly" on the hub of the needle and suture it to the skin. An injection cap is placed on the needle, and a small amount of warmed saline should be injected to check the patency. (you may do this prior to securing the catheter).

9) Flush the needle with heparinized solution. An additional bandage material is used to protect the catheter and leg.

10) For ulnar placement, the bird should be anesthetized, and the feathers of the dorsal and distal ulna plucked from the area of the wrist joint. This joint is just proximal to the superficial ulnar artery and superficial digital flexor tendon, which are visible through the skin as landmarks.

11) The skin should be surgically prepped and the insertion area infiltrated with dilute lidocaine.

12) Support the wing with one hand, and with the other, position an appropriately sized needle at the distal end of the ulna, parallel to the diaphysis. Drive it carefully into the medullary canal using firm pressure and a slight twisting motion.

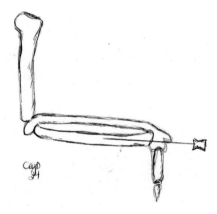

Figure 21.9 Interosseous catheterization of the ulna, showing the insertion site.

13) Once the needle penetrates the cortex, it then passes without resistance in the marrow cavity. To check, aspirate using a syringe to draw a small amount of the marrow into the needle hub.

14) If resistance is met during the insertion, it is likely the needle is crossing another cortex, and it should be withdrawn slightly and redirected.

15) Once seated, attach an injection cap, and inject a small amount of the fluid watching the basilic vein where the bolus can be seen. Alternatively, radiographs can confirm correct positioning.

16) Flush the needle with heparinized solution. Secure by making a "butterfly" of tape around the hub and suture it to the skin. Then, use a light figure-of-eight bandage to immobilize the wing.

17) Administration of fluids or other medications through the intraosseous catheters can cause intense pain if there is much pressure, so small volumes delivered slowly are necessary. It is recommended that the largest syringe to be used is 3 mL to minimize pressure delivery.

Rationale/Amplification

Oral administration is preferred in birds with only mild dehydration, provided they are not vomiting and that they do not have crop/gastrointestinal stasis.
Parenteral fluids are often started with subcutaneous (SC) administration while the bird is prepared for further diagnostics, catheter placement, and stabilization.
Absorption from subcutaneous in the inguinal (precrural fold), sub/interscapular area, or axillary areas is usually rapid – within 15 minutes. Many psittacines may develop edema from large volumes. SC fluids are poorly absorbed during severe dehydration and hypovolemic shock.
IV fluids may be difficult as their administration means continuous restraint or sedation/anesthesia.
Indwelling catheters may not be tolerated in smaller birds.
Intravenous fluids are often given as a one-off bolus or set up as continuous infusion in an anesthetized bird by using a syringe infusion pump.
If a bird is severely dehydrated and cannot tolerate handling for one-off IV bolus, it should be placed in a warm, humid environment with SC fluids until it is stabile that an IO catheter can be placed under sedation and local anesthesia.
The route and volume need to be calculated per each case.
During surgery, fluids are generally given at a rate of 10 mL/kg/h.
Perioperative subcutaneous fluids are usually given at 5% of body weight q 12–24 hours.
Dehydration correction follows similar rules to that used in mammals – percent dehydration added to the assumed 50–100 mL/kg/24 hours.
Complications of intraosseous catheters can be osteomyelitis if left in place for more than 72 hours. If the bird is osteoporotic, the placement may fracture the bone. Placement in laying female birds with hyperostotic bones may be impossible due to the lack of a medullary canal.

Syringe pumps: A syringe pump is useful in delivering a steady volume rather than a bolus. This provides consistent delivery overtime and can be adjusted to deliver the calculated volume per time unit. For continuous fluid therapy, such as in surgeries or in prolonged hospitalization, a syringe pump can provide a good option. Although it minimizes staff time in some ways, a designated staff person must still continually monitor the pump, the infusion line, and the infusion site for signs of obstruction, leakage, or catheter disengagement. There are a number of commercially available pumps, many which utilize small volume syringes that work well for many pet birds less than 1–2 kgs.

BIBLIOGRAPHY

Doneley B. Clinical techniques. In: *Avian Medicine and Surgery in Practice. Companion and Aviary Birds*. 2011. Manson Publishing Ltd/The Veterinary Press, London, UK. pp 55–68.

Schnellbacher R, Beaufrère H. Catheterization and venipuncture. In: Graham JE, Doss GA, Beaufrère H (eds). *Exotic Animal Emergency and Critical Care Medicine*. 2021. John Wiley & Sons, Inc, Hoboken, NJ. pp 1147–1166.

22

Positioning for Imaging

Imaging is most commonly done with radiographs, although more advanced imaging techniques such as CT or MRI are being used for more detailed, specific conditions. Ultrasonography is useful particularly for cardiac, liver, and general abdominal imaging.

Use of general anesthesia is a choice of the clinician, dependent largely on the bird's temperament and clinical condition; however, the use of midazolam intranasally at 2 mg/kg provides safe relaxation, enough for most radiographic procedures. CT and MRI scan require full anesthesia as the bird may need to be held still for extended periods of time. Ultrasonography rarely needs anesthesia, although light sedation may be useful particularly for cardiac examinations that may take longer than 15 minutes.

Contrast studies are frequently done, primarily to assess the gastrointestinal tract, although localized contrast can be done in other tissues and systems.

Many birds can be positioned with the use of acrylic boards that have ties and straps that hold the head, legs, and wings while awake. These boards are available commercially and make it fairly easy to get accurate, symmetrical positioning with no damage to the feathers or the bird. They also do not inhibit respirations. However, they may not work for birds under 100 grams. Frequently the cassette itself will serve as the platform and the bird positioned using a nonadhesive tape (such as a masking tape which does not damage the feathers) and small sandbags or weighted protective gloves.

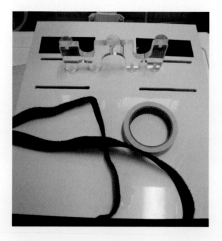

Figure 22.1 An acrylic avian positioning board and straps and tape that are used to secure the bird.

Manual of Clinical Procedures in Pet Birds, First Edition. Cathy A. Johnson-Delaney and Tracy Bennett.
© 2025 John Wiley & Sons, Inc. Published 2025 by John Wiley & Sons, Inc.
Companion website: www.wiley.com/go/johnson-delaney/manual

Points to consider with avian radiography and positioning.

1) Because there is no diaphragm, the heart is in contact with the gastrointestinal tract and liver. The heart and liver appear fused on the ventrodorsal project are are referred to as the cardiohepatic silhouette.
2) The viscera within the coelom was compacted due to the presence of air sacs, and it can be difficult to assess individual organs.
3) There is rarely much fat surrounding organs, unlike mammals, so it further reduces the ability to distinguish organs. Avian fat has radio-opacity similar to many soft tissues.

Procedure

Ventrodorsal (VD) view positioning (for radiography, CT, and MRI)

Purpose

To obtain a symmetrical, straight-line position with the bird in dorsal recumbency. This position also is used for the skull, with the head extended using a small string, wire loop, or gauze strip.

Complications

- If the bird is not sedated or anesthetized, getting the exact positioning can be difficult, as the bird may wiggle, especially when taped or velcroed into position.

Equipment

- Radiograph, cassettes, and digital computer/software
- Restraint board or surface to tape the bird in position.
- Masking tape
- Sandbags of various sizes
- If sedation or anesthesia to be used – medications and anesthesia machine.

Technical Action

1) Place the bird on its back with the head and neck extended cranially. Fasten the head/neck restraint device or lay strips of the masking tape across the neck.

Figure 22.2 A   Diagram of positioning.

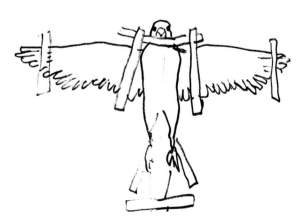

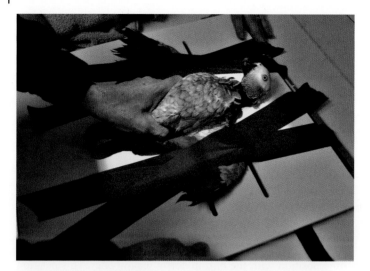

Figure 22.2 B Actual bird shown placed in proper positioning.

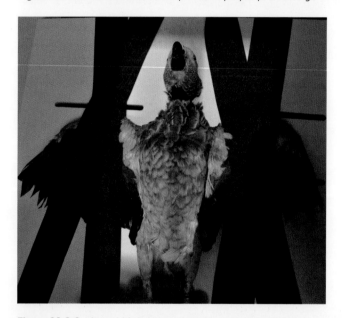

Figure 22.2 C Actual bird shown placed in proper positioning.

2) The sternum (keel) bone must be perfectly aligned so that it is superimposed over the spinal column.
3) The wings are usually extended laterally, symmetrically, and taped or secured.
4) The legs are extended caudally and should be parallel to each other. Secure with a tape or ties.
5) The center of the radiographic beam should be at the center of the bird or the center of whatever structure you are primarily examining.

Rationale/Amplification

1: This can also be done easily as a standing ventrodorsal position, with the bird vertical. It requires a radiographic head able to rotate for standing laterals.

2: if this is not superimposed, it indicates body rotation, making it difficult to assess the cardio-hepatic size or evaluate other organs.

Procedure

Laterolateral (LL) view positioning (for radiography, CT, and MRI)

Purpose

To obtain a perfect lateral view of the body, with the wings stretched dorsally and superimposed on each other. The shoulders should be superimposed on each other. If the case requires separate views of the wings, these may be taken after the full body, and the wings are separated. The wings should have a thick pad placed between them to maintain both parallel to the surface. The legs should be extended ventrocaudally, with hips and legs superimposed on each other. A small pad can be used to keep the legs parallel to the surface. If a separate view of the legs is needed, then the legs can be separated. Indicate which foot is forward. Generally, birds are placed on the right side unless pathology exists to position on the left side. This position can also be used for the skull, preferably straightening the neck and extending the skull using a small string, wire loop, or gauze strip. Keeping the cervical spine straight may require a small pad placed in the mid-cervical spine.

Complications

- If the bird is not sedated or anesthetized, getting the exact positioning can be difficult, as the bird may wiggle, especially when taped or velcroed into position.

Equipment

- Radiograph, cassettes, and digital computer/software
- Restraint board or surface to tape the bird in position
- Masking tape
- Sand bags of various sizes
- If sedation or anesthesia to be used — medications and anesthesia machine

Technical Action

1) Place the bird on its right side with the head and neck extended cranially. Fasten the head/neck restraint device or lay strips of the masking tape across the neck.

Figure 22.3 A Diagram of the lateral position.

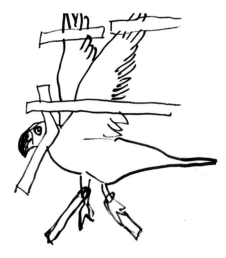

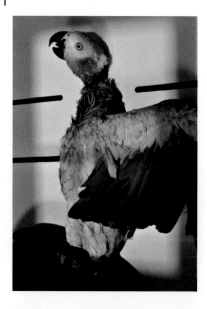

Figure 22.3 B Actual bird in position for a lateral radiograph.

2) The shoulders should be superimposed over each other.
3) The wings are usually extended dorsally and superimposed (use a pad between the wings to keep them parallel to the table surface). If this is not done, the body may rotate when the left (upper) wing is stretched out. Avoid excessive tension on the extension of the wings as it can impede respiration.
4) The legs are extended ventrocaudally and should be parallel to each other. Secure with tape or ties.
5) If views of the hips are needed, the upper leg is stretched outward, allowing good visualization of the contralateral hip. To view the other hip, the bird will need to be repositioned on its other side.
6) The center of the radiographic beam should be at the center of the bird or the center of whatever structure you are primarily examining.
7) If the machine in use has the capability of rotation of the beam, then a standing lateral view can be done. Positioning is still done as above, but with the bird standing next to the plate. The masking tape is usually used to secure the wings, neck, and/or legs as needed. In emergencies, this view can be done quickly with the bird in normal standing position – a quick screening process for the presence of heavy metals, retained eggs, and some fractures, especially of the wings or legs.

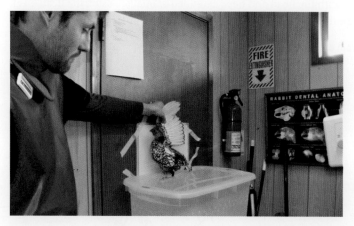

Figure 22.4 This is demonstrating positioning for a standing lateral. Before exposure, the wings would be taped into place, and the radiology technician would step back from the patient to a safe distance so that he/she is not exposed to the beam or scatter.

Rationale/Amplification

\# 1: If the clinical condition warrants, the LL position can be done with the left side down.

\# 2: If this is not superimposed, it indicates body rotation, making it difficult to assess the lungs, spine, and viscera.

Procedure

Radiographic positioning of the wing

Purpose

To obtain two views (lateral and VD) of the wing. This is usually described as mediolaterally and caudocranially.

Complications

- To get the caudocranial view, the positioning requires the wing be rotated so that the primary feathers are pointed vertically to the beam.

Equipment

- Radiograph, cassettes, and digital computer/software
- Restraint board or surface to tape the bird in position.
- Masking tape or cord ties long enough to extend the wing and position vertically.
- Sandbags of various sizes
- If sedation or anesthesia to be used – medications and anesthesia machine.

Technical Action

1) Place the bird on its side with the wing to be examined. The wing can be extended dorsally. The other wing can be placed extended but caudal to the other wing. Fasten the head/neck restraint device or lay strips of the masking tape across the neck.
2) The shoulders should be superimposed over each other.
3) Avoid excessive tension on the extension of the wings as it can impede respiration.
4) The legs are extended ventrocaudally and should be parallel to each other. Secure with tape or ties.
5) The center of the radiographic beam should be centered over the portion of the wing to be evaluated. This will provide the mediolateral view.
6) To obtain the cranial–caudal or caudocranial view, the bird must be repositioned (usually in the VD position, again with the keel superimposed over the spin) so that the pathologic wing can be extended out from the body and rotated so that the feathers point vertical to the beam. This is more difficult to position with tape or ties and in some cases must be manually held with the operator in leaded gown and gloves, holding the wing tip.
7) The beam should be centered over the section of the wing to be examined.

Rationale/Amplification

\# 1: If there is a presumed fracture, all wing extensions and manipulations must be done with utmost care to prevent further dislocation and damage. Perfect views may not be possible due to the injury, but an attempt should still be made to get two views.

\# 2: If this is not superimposed, it indicates body rotation, making it difficult to assess structures.

Procedure

Contrast radiography

Purpose

To outline various organs for visualization of the structure and function

Complications

- If the proper amount of contrast media is not used, it may be difficult to assess.
- The bird should be starved so that there is a more empty GI tract.

Equipment

- Anesthesia agents of choice
- Radiographic equipment
- Restraint equipment, e.g. towels and radiographic restraint board
- Appropriate sized feeding tube to deliver contrast media into the crop (GI study)
- Barium sulfate (25–45% commercial solution): use 20 mg/kg. Do not use for suspected GI rupture
- Iohexol (250 mg/mL solution): use 10 mL/kg delivered by gavage for GI

Technical Action

1) Restrain the bird in a towel and deliver the contrast media by gavage into the crop.
2) Immediately take VD and lateral radiographs. (note, the bird can be anesthetized for this whole procedure, although it is advised that the bird be held vertically, possibly intubated to prevent regurgitation of contrast media. General anesthesia does not affect the GI transit time).
3) Time intervals for views: 0, 30, 60, and 120 minutes (although this can vary per patient and problem).
4) Most birds will not be anesthetized for all these views!

Rationale/Amplification

1: Gavage is necessary to deliver the full amount of the contrast media. It is best to hold the bird upright during this process and as much as possible throughout the study. In between shots, allow the bird to be in its home cage or perch.

Procedure

Positioning for ultrasonography

Purpose

To provide access for ultrasonography to coelomic viscera and the heart. For liver and cardiac assessment, the probe is placed just caudal and dorsal to the keel, pointing craniad. The liver serves as the window to the heart. Refer to Chapter 16 on positioning for cardiac ultrasound.

Complications

- Feathers and air sacs, which impede the ultrasonic beam. Feathers are wetted with alcohol and/ or ultrasound gel, but still may create artifacts due to the small amount of calcification within them. For detailed cardiac examination, it may be necessary to pluck a few feathers just distal to the sternum.

Equipment

- Restraint equipment (e.g. towels and restraint strap)
- Ultrasonographic unit and probe with a small window
- Ultrasound gel
- Isopropyl alcohol
- Gauze sponges

Technical Action

1) Restrain the bird in an upright position.
2) Apply a small amount of alcohol and/or ultrasonic gel to the skin just caudal to the sternum.
3) Angle the probe to scan cranially. For other organs, the probe can be moved on the midline, fanned, and angled as needed.
4) After scanning is completed, wipe off all gel/alcohol so that the feathers are clean and dry.

Rationale/Amplification

1: It is easier to view the heart in the upright position, as the bird is less stressed and has more normal respirations.

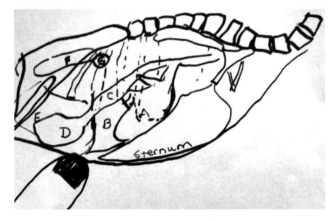

Figure 22.5   Diagram of the position for placement of the ultrasound probe. A: Heart; B: Liver, C: Proventriculus; D: Ventriculus; E: Cloaca, intestines; F: Kidney; G: Gonad.

BIBLIOGRAPHY

Crosta L, Melillo A, Schnitzer P. Basic radiography. In: Chitty J, Monks D (eds). *BSAVA Manual of Avian Practice*. 2018. BSAVA, Quedgeley, UK. pp 269–285.

Lennox AM, Crosta L, Buerke M. The effects of isoflurane anesthesia on gastrointestinal transit time. 2002. Proceedings of the 23rd AAV Annual Conference, pp. 53–55.

23

Euthanasia Techniques

While methods for avian euthanasia from the AVMA Guidelines for Euthanasia, 2020, describe acceptable methods for birds including poultry, laboratory, wildlife, eggs, and chicks, there are only a few methods that are acceptable for pet birds, particularly if the owner wishes to be present. All methods should render a bird unconscious with no pain or anxiety and should bring about a gentle death. If the bird is to be submitted for necropsy and histopathology, certain methods may be preferred by the pathologist to minimize artifacts.

It is highly recommended that all birds receive anti-anxiety and analgesia medications along with sedation prior to the actual agent used for euthanasia. It may be advantageous to place an intravenous catheter in some of the larger birds, or if the bird was critically ill, it may already have an interosseous catheter. While the AVMA Euthanasia Guidelines 2020 (Table 23.1) discuss intra-celomic injections, for pet birds, this is usually not done. The reason it is not considered acceptable in the presence of the owner is that giving an injection into the body is objectionable to the owner, and it also carries the potential of pain, hitting an organ, causing internal bleeding, injecting into an air sac which may prolong the euthanasia solution taking effect and just the variability in absorption and effectiveness. Most pet birds are given sedative/anxiolytic/analgesics by injection – either IM, IN, or IV, and then the euthanasia solution is delivered IV, or the bird is euthanized by inhalant anesthesia.

Although intracardiac injections are listed in the AVMA Euthanasia Guidelines, this is considered a very painful event and if used should be done only after verifying the bird is in unrecoverable deep anesthesia, usually in respiratory arrest and possibly in fibrillation, just to hasten full cardiac arrest. In the author's opinion, this should not be done in the owner's presence as it can be distressing to the owner in visualizing a needle going into the heart. Accessing the avian heart is through the "v" shape in the cranial sternum, through the crop and great vessels. Ultrasound guidance can be used to confirm needle access and cardiac arrest.

The decision to euthanize the bird must be made with the owner. Most veterinarians will work with an owner to rehome a healthy bird that the owner requested euthanasia only because they can no longer keep it. The welfare and quality of life of the bird must be considered when there is a clinical condition.

If the owner wishes to be present, the steps of the euthanasia process should be discussed, including the stages of relaxation, the possibility of a moment of excitement, and then how death with be determined – if by a stethoscope or in many cases, Electrocardiogram (ECG).

Manual of Clinical Procedures in Pet Birds, First Edition. Cathy A. Johnson-Delaney and Tracy Bennett.
© 2025 John Wiley & Sons, Inc. Published 2025 by John Wiley & Sons, Inc.
Companion website: www.wiley.com/go/johnson-delaney/manual

Table 23.1 AVMA guidelines for Euthanasia 2020 applicable for individual pet birds.

Method	Agent	Application	Comments
Inhalant	Isoflurane, sevoflurane, and halothane	In chamber, by face mask, or if already anesthetized and intubated, by endotracheal administration	A bird should be administered a sedative with anxiolytic properties (e.g. midazolam) along with other injectable agents such as an analgesic prior to the administration of the inhalant. This decreases fear and stress. This may be used as an anesthetic prior to the IV administration of a euthanasia agent (e.g. sodium pentobarbital) or as the sole euthanasia agent itself, administered at high concentration.
	Carbon dioxide	High concentration (>40%), in a chamber. This is not appropriate for neonatal birds as they are more acclimated to high CO_2 concentrations	Bird should be heavily sedated and preferably wrapped in a towel so that unconscious involuntary motor activity like wing flapping does not occur.
Injection	Barbiturate: (e.g. sodium pentobarbital) Note: These agents are normally delivered IV, as they are alkaline and can be irritating and painful if injected directly into tissues	Intracelomic injection	Do not inject into air sacs, which could cause drowning or expose the respiratory system to irritating agents. The bird should be fully anesthetized prior to this route.
		Intraosseous – tibia	Do not use this route in femur/humerus as pneumatic bones communicate directly with the respiratory system. The bird should be fully anesthetized prior to this route.
		Intracardiac	Only to be used if the bird is fully unconscious or anesthetized.
		Intravenous	Preferable to have the bird sedated and calm prior to administration by the intravenous route. Catheter in the leg or wing in larger species may ease administration. The bird should be wrapped in a towel or held such that it cannot flap its wings during euthanasia.
	Potassium chloride	Intravenous or Intracardiac	Administration only if a bird is unconscious or completely anesthetized prior to injection.

(Continued)

Table 23.1 (Continued)

Method	Agent	Application	Comments
Adjunctive methods			
	Exsanguination	Blood collected through a catheter or intracardiac	Only acceptable if the bird is unconscious or fully anesthetized and if a large blood sample is needed for diagnostics or research.
	Thoracic compression	Manual compression	Only acceptable if the bird is unconscious or fully anesthetized with an injectable agent prior to compression. Not recommended.
Unacceptable			
	Thoracic compression	Manual compression	Do not use on an awake, conscious bird. This is considered extremely stressful, inducing fear and panic, while physically painful.
Special considerations: eggs, embryos, and neonates			
Perform based on best available data and assure that conscious suffering does not occur	Embryo at >80% incubation	Methods as described above for neonates	Anesthetic overdose and prolonged (>20 min) exposure to CO_2.
	Eggs < 80% incubation	Research is still evolving as to acceptable methods	Prolonged exposure (>20 min) to CO_2, cooling (<4 °C for 4 h) or freezing.

Equipment

- Stethoscope and/or other monitoring equipment
- Restraint equipment such as a towel
- Alcohol for wetting the feathers and exposing the vein.
- Appropriately sized needles and syringes.
- Pre-euthanasia sedatives: intranasal administration of butorphanol at 2 mg/kg and midazolam at 2 mg/kg provides good sedation and pain control for most pet birds.
- Intravenous catheter such as 24 or 26 ga, plus plug, and tape for securing.
- Euthanasia solution: pentobarbital primarily.
- Anesthesia machine with inhalants such as isoflurane and appropriate size mask or chamber.

Procedure

Euthanasia by injection

Purpose

To euthanize the bird with an intravenous or intraosseous injection of a barbiturate euthanasia solution.

Complications

- Venous or intraosseous access may be difficult in very small birds. An intraosseous catheter placement is considered painful and is done as a procedure (see Chapter 21). The basilic vein is an easily accessible vein; however, it tends to be fragile and will cause a hematoma, and the exit from the vein must be held for several minutes following the solution administration. The tibio-tarsal vein is accessible in birds heavier than 200 grams. Small birds may have the euthanasia solution injection via the jugular vein after the bird is heavily sedated.

Technical Action

1) Gently restrain the bird in a towel.
2) Give intranasal butorphanol/midazolam.
3) When the bird is relaxed and somewhat sleepy:
4) Lay the bird in dorsal recumbency on a warmed surface and extend a wing.
5) Wet the surface over the ventral elbow where the basilic vein is visible.
6) Have an assistant apply gentle digital pressure medially to enlarge the vein.
7) If a catheter is to be inserted, it can be done, capped, and taped in place.
8) Euthanasia solution can be administered through the catheter.
9) If no catheter is placed, then the needle can be inserted directly into the vein. The assistant should release the digital pressure, and slow injection of the euthanasia solution is done.
10) Remove the needle and apply digital pressure at the injection site to prevent bleeding. A piece of cotton or gauze can be used under the finger on the site.
11) If the basilic vein is too small, the tibiotarsal vein in larger birds is an alternative. The jugular vein is available in small birds and is usually not catheterized. Injection is directly through a needle inserted into the vein.
12) Gently roll the bird over into a sternal position and observe.
13) Verify death via a stethoscope (or by instrumentation).
14) The author usually says something like "goodbye (bird's name)" and pats the bird gently. Leave the room and allow the owner some time with the bird.
15) If they are taking the bird's body home with them, it is advisable to wrap the bird in a towel or cloth that they have brought, enclose the bird in double zipper closing plastic bags, wrap in another cloth, and place in a box. Remove any catheters and bandages if present. If the vein leaks when the catheter is pulled, clean the area, and tape on a cotton ball over the vein. Some clinics offer footprints on a card to go home. Be sure the owners know to leave the bird in the bags and bury deeply so that wild predators do not dig the bird up.
16) If the bird is to be necropsied: remove to the laboratory for the procedure.
17) If the bird is to be cremated, when the owners have said their goodbyes, remove the bird in the towel to be processed for the cremation services.

Procedure

Inhalation euthanasia

Technical Action

1) Gently restrain the bird in a towel.
2) Give intranasal butorphanol/midazolam.
3) When the bird is relaxed and somewhat sleepy:
4) Lay the bird in sternal recumbency on a warmed surface.
5) Apply an appropriately sized mask over the bird's beak and nares.
6) Start inhalant anesthesia on the highest setting on the vaporizer, with oxygen and/or nitrous oxide.
7) Monitor respirations and heart rate.
8) Usually, the bird will go into respiratory arrest within a few minutes; cardiac arrest may take a few more minutes.
9) Verify death via a stethoscope (or by instrumentation).
10) Usually, the owner is waiting in a grief or exam room. Bring the bird wrapped loosely in the towel back to the owners to say goodbye.
11) The author usually says something like "goodbye (bird's name)" and pats the bird gently. Leave the room and allow the owner some time with the bird.
12) If they are taking the bird's body home with them, it is advisable to wrap the bird in a towel or cloth that they have brought, enclose the bird in double zipper closing plastic bags, wrap in another cloth, and place in a box. Some clinics offer footprints on a card to go home.
13) If the bird is to be necropsied: remove to the laboratory for the procedure.
14) If the bird is to be cremated, when the owners have said their goodbyes, remove the bird in the towel to be processed for the cremation services.

BIBLIOGRAPHY

AVMA *Guidelines for the Euthanasia of Animals* 2020 Edition. S5 Avians, Schaumberg, IL, USA. Pp 79–82.

Chitty J, Monks D. Euthanasia of birds. In: Chitty J, Monks D. (eds). *BSAVA Manual of Avian Practice. A Foundation Manual*. 2018. BSAVA, Quedgeley, UK. Pg 231.

Montesinos A. Basic techniques. In: Chitty J, Monks D (eds). *BSAVA Manual of Avian Practice. A Foundation Manual*. 2018. BSAVA, Quedgeley, UK. pp 215–231.

24

Analgesia, Sedation, and Anesthesia: Medications and Procedures

Providing relief from pain and stress can begin in the examination room. When it is perceived that a bird is in pain, or it is severely anxious, frantic, and frightened, administration of an analgesic coupled with a sedative will not only provide relief to the bird but will allow the clinician to better examine and formulate a diagnostic and treatment plan for that bird. Pain is usually categorized as acute or chronic, but relief initially may be provided by the same medication. Clinical assessment of the degree of pain exhibited by the bird's physical and mental demeanor is beyond the scope of this text. The clinician must also quickly evaluate the perceived level of anxiety and fear and choose a combination of medications that may be of quick benefit.

With many of the drugs now having had pharmacologic studies done in pet bird species, and many referred papers listing acceptable drugs and combinations to achieve analgesia, relaxation, or sedation, a practitioner needs to develop protocols based on the science along with experience. When an analgesic and sedative agent is administered, diagnostic testing can be done more efficiently, quickly, and a therapy plan initiated. An awake, struggling bird can make getting a good blood draw, diagnostic radiographs, and other diagnostics difficult, not to mention causing more stress and potential injury not only to the bird but also to the hospital staff. It may make any disease condition worse.

Many texts cite the use of butorphanol and midazolam, in combination, to facilitate the examination and diagnostic testing and for initiation of therapy. The combination can also be used as a pre-anesthetic. Just "masking a bird down" without pre-medications is not considered best practices any longer, as it has been shown that there can be extreme fluctuations in catecholamines, corticosteroids, blood pressure, and other parameters, which can cause risk under general anesthesia in addition to making regulation more difficult.

The term "multi-modal" analgesia/anesthesia is now considered best practice. By using different drugs for different parts of the analgesia/sedation/anesthesia, lower doses and concentrations of all can be used and the bird maintained on a more stable plane of anesthesia, with faster recovery time. Use of reversal agents is also common.

While a bird is under the influence of sedation or anesthesia, it needs to be monitored. A staff member should be assigned per case to attend to the bird and monitor vitals at specific intervals. All of this care needs to be recorded in the medical record.

Before administering these medications, the owner needs to be informed of the action of the drugs and the rationale for using them on their bird. A signed consent form should be entered into the medical record. If a bird is to be sent home on an analgesic that may have sedative properties, it is advantageous to administer the first dose in the hospital to observe for side effects. Owners need also be counseled on adjusting the bird's caging and furnishings to provide easy access to food and water and decrease any potential for falling or trauma within the cage.

Routes of administration of drugs are described in Chapters 3 and 4.

Procedure

Providing analgesia

Purpose

Administration of an analgesic to alleviate pain.

Complications

- The exact dose for that species may not have been studied, so dosing is based on similar species.
- Metabolic compromise can alter drug metabolism and either increase or decrease the effects and/or side effects.
- Assessment of effectiveness is often anecdotal and may rely on the owner's observations of behavior.

Equipment

- Analgesics (e.g. butorphanol, buprenorphine, and hydromorphone,)
- If the drug to be used is a controlled substance, then regulatory paperwork must be completed per law.
- Nonsteroidal anti-inflammatory drugs (NSAIDS) can also provide analgesia and decrease inflammation, without many of the sedation side effects. They may not be strong enough alone for the level of pain but can be combined with opioids.
- Formulary
- Scale and calculator
- Various sizes syringes and needles
- Restraint equipment (e.g. towel)
- Oxygen via face mask if needed.
- Warming cage, incubator, or critical care housing if necessary
- Reversal agent if available, as necessary

Technical Action

1) The bird should be weighed upon removal from its cage or carrier, usually at the beginning of the office visit.
2) From observation, initial physical examination, estimate the level of pain and choose an analgesic agent(s).
3) Draw up the analgesic to be given – in the appropriate delivery system.
4) Gently restrain the bird in a towel, administer the agent, and allow the bird to go back in its carrier or cage while the drug takes effect.

Figure 24.1 Restrained bird receiving an IM injection.

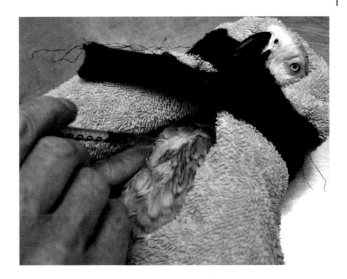

5) Once it seems the bird is less painful, the examination and procedures can be continued.

Rationale/Amplification

4–5: If the bird exhibits too much sedation, opioid administration can be reversed using naloxone. This can occur if the bird is metabolically compromised or dehydrated or if the dose range may be incorrect for that species.

Procedure

Providing sedation

Purpose

To provide sedation, relaxation, decrease anxiety, and decrease fear. Sedation can accompany provision of analgesia. The combination can be used as a pre-anesthetic, or to facilitate examination, diagnostic testing, and as part of a treatment regimen.

Complications

- Pharmacologic data for each species of pet bird are not available, so dosing is based on a closely related species or sized bird. Dose ranges may be too high or too low and may need adjustment.
- Excessive sedation will require supportive care: ventilation, monitoring, warming, oxygen, and even agent reversal.
- Depending on the underlying disease and metabolic state, levels of sedation may not be at the level predicted and have a different duration of action than desired.

Equipment

- Sedatives such as a benzodiazepine (e.g. diazepam and midazolam)

- If the drug to be used is a controlled substance, then regulatory paperwork must be completed per law.
- Gabapentin has multiple functions but at some doses may be anxiolytic and cause sedation.
- Combinations of butorphanol and midazolam are commonly used for sedation – for examinations, diagnostic testing, and as pre-anesthetics.
- Formulary
- Scale and calculator
- Various sizes syringes and needles
- Restraint equipment (e.g. towel)
- Oxygen via a face mask if needed.

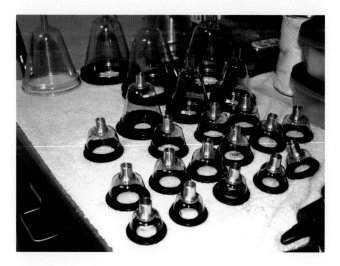

Figure 24.2   A variety of types and sizes of masks should be available.

- Warming cage, incubator, or critical care housing if necessary
- Reversal agent if available, as necessary

Technical Action

1) The bird should be weighed upon removal from its cage or carrier, usually at the beginning of the office visit.
2) From observation at initial physical examination, estimate the sedation level desired. Note: an analgesic may also be given in combination if pain is present.
3) Draw up the sedative to be given – in the appropriate delivery system.
4) Gently restrain the bird in a towel, administer the agent, and allow the bird to go back in its carrier or cage while the drug takes effect.
5) Once it seems the bird is less active, anxious, and is sedate, i.e. slightly sleepy, the examination and procedures can be continued.

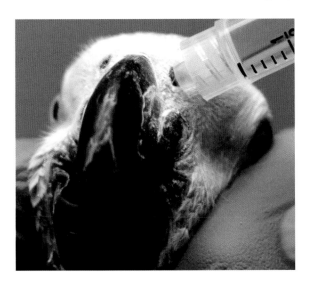

Figure 24.3 Bird receiving an intranasal dose of a sedative.

Rationale/Amplification

4–5: If the bird exhibits too much sedation, benzodiazepines can be reversed with flumazenil. Opioids can be reversed using naloxone. This can occur if the bird is metabolically compromised, ill, or dehydrated, or if the dose range may be incorrect for that species.

Procedure

Local anesthesia

Purpose

Produce regional analgesia and anesthesia by blocking the transmission of noxious impulses. Local blocking can be done pre-operatively to prevent pain at surgery or injection sites and used in conjunction with general sedation or anesthesia. Local anesthetic usage is part of a multimodal approach and usually allows for decreased levels of general anesthesia. Bupivacaine and lidocaine act by blocking sodium channels in the nerve axon that interferes with action conduction potentials along the nerve.

There are three basic types of administration of local anesthetics:

a) Regional infiltration from injection in/around the area to be anesthetized. This includes intra-articular and intralesional.
b) Incision line infiltration.
c) Splash blocks – where the anesthetic is sprayed/irrigated into an area.

Complications

- In small birds, local or topical anesthetics used particularly in the eyes or sinuses may cause profound central nervous system depression if passed into the brain due to the site of application.
- Birds have thin skin and little subcutaneous fat, so subcutaneous and dermal administration of agents may not dissipate and cover the area as well as in mammals.

- Overdosing of lidocaine may cause seizures and death in small birds. Other toxic side effects can include tremors, seizures, ataxia, stupor, recumbency, cardiovascular effects, and death.
- Lidocaine has a fairly short duration of action (1–3 hours), and bupivacaine may last for 4–10 hours based on duration in mammals. In birds, it may be a shorter duration for both agents.

Equipment

- Restraint equipment (e.g. towel)
- Formulary
- Scale and calculator
- Surgical preparation solution (such as 2% chlorhexidine surgical scrub solution)
- Gauze sponges
- 25–27 ga needles, usually on insulin or tuberculin 1 cc syringe
- Lidocaine 1 or 2% or bupivacaine. Usually, the dosage is diluted further at least 1:10 for birds
- Lidocaine dose: 1–4 mg/kg; dilute 1:10 with sterile water; do not exceed 4 mg/kg.
- Bupivacaine maximum dose: 1 mg/kg. May also dilute with sterile water.

Technical Action

1) Restrain the bird in a towel with the area to be anesthetized exposed.
2) Note: the bird can already be sedated or anesthetized for the local anesthetic to be administered as part of a pre-operative preparation, or it can be done in the awake, restrained bird for an awake small procedure.
3) Clean the skin or lesion site with surgical scrub as done to prepare a surgery site.
4) Administer the calculated dosage to the area. For cutaneous mass removals, circumferential infiltration along with intralesional injection can be done.
5) Dab any bleeding and dry the area/feathers around the site with a gauze. (Remember that wet feathers can cool the bird – an undesirable effect.)
6) Proceed with the surgery or other procedure.

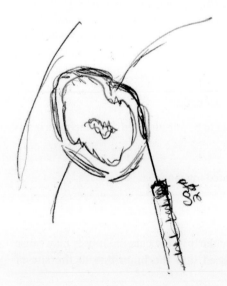

Figure 24.4 Administration of a local anesthetic around a lesion. Inject a small amount of the local anesthetic around the mass, creating overlapping bubbles/blebs of fluid.

Rationale/Amplification

4: Do not exceed the calculated maximum dosage per body weight. Consider the anatomical site and location of innervation. Avoid injections into blood vessels. Transilluminating a lesion may show major blood vessels, particularly in a tumor. Let the owner know that there can be bruising at the injection sites.

Procedure

General anesthesia

Purpose

Induce a state of unconsciousness and cessation of pain or perception of noxious stimuli.

This can be done by using several methods or combinations of methods: constant rate infusion or intravenous injection, inhalation (most commonly used), and/or intramuscular injections. General anesthesia should be preceded by analgesia/sedative administration to decrease fright, spiking of blood pressure and endogenous corticosterone release, and other metabolic parameter disruptions that can alter the amount of the anesthetic to be delivered, as well as evaluation of depth.

Complications

- Decreased ventilation as most birds are in dorsal recumbency and gravity plus anesthesia decrease sternal excursion during breathing. Positive pressure ventilation is indicated to counteract this decreased respiratory effort.
- Inadequate skill and training of the team monitoring the anesthetic state of the bird. This includes use of equipment such as ECG, pulse oximetry, capnography, cloacal thermometry, and direct observation. Pupillary reflex, palpebral reflexes, and other indicators of depth may not be as reliable as in mammals.
- Underlying disease processes may not be fully explored prior to the anesthesia (especially if a surgical procedure and coelomic exploration are performed).
- Avian full general anesthesia is usually kept to as short a duration as possible. In the author's experience, longer than 30 minutes may result in increased risk of prolonged recovery and/ or death.
- If during anesthesia the depth is too deep, immediate cessation or decrease in agent administration must be done. (see Chapter 20).

Equipment

- Restraint equipment (e.g. towel)
- Formulary
- Scale and calculator
- Anesthetic agents to be used: injectable inhalant (see Table 24.3 Anesthetic Drugs)
- Needles/syringes appropriate for the size of the bird and method of drug administration
- Masks, endotracheal tubes (prefer uncuffed, can use other types of catheters, modified French tubes for birds smaller than 100 grams), material for tying/securing the endotracheal tube and holding the beak open so that the tube is not compressed, and breath can be visualized. Oral mucous membranes must be visible.

- Monitoring equipment: ECG, thermal, pulse oximetry, (side-stream) capnography sensor, audio Doppler, stethoscope, respirometer, blood pressure cuffs, and sphygmomanometer.
- Tape to secure various sensors
- Warming system
- Fluid administration (see Chapter 21)

Technical Action

1) Restrain the bird and administer pre-anesthetic analgesic-sedative agents.
2) When the bird is deemed calm, sedated, begin the administration of the next agent to induce unconsciousness and loss of jaw (beak) tone to allow for intubation. This includes using a mask with an inhalation anesthetic agent delivered with oxygen.
3) The bird should be laying on a warming system during induction.
4) When sufficiently relaxed, open the beak (usually done with a soft speculum or by having an assistant open the beak, using the fingers, or with gauze strips to pull it open gently.
5) Observe the glottis and pass a noncuffed tube of appropriate width into the glottis. Secure the tube with elastic or gauze strips or other materials to prevent the tube from exiting the glottis or extending further down the trachea.
6) Connect the bird to an inhalant anesthesia machine of the inhalant to be used. If anesthesia is to be delivered via intravenous or intraosseous infusion, then place a larger mask covering the head of the bird for flow-by oxygen delivery.

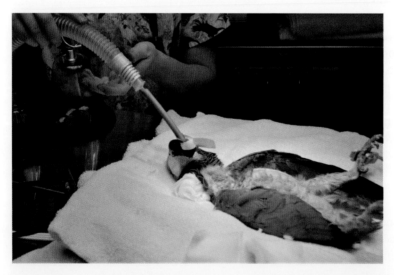

Figure 24.5 Anesthetized, intubated bird on a warming blanket, with pulse oximetry probe attached.

7) Attach the monitoring equipment and begin recording vitals at frequent intervals – usually every 5 minutes. Visual observation of the patient by the designated anesthetist or nurse is constant, and the state of the patient is communicated to the surgeon.
8) Deliver anesthetic agents to achieve a surgical depth of anesthesia – where reflexes and stimulus from pain are absent.
9) When surgery/procedure is completed, stop inhalant agent delivery and leave the bird on oxygen. If injectable anesthetics are used, administer reversal agents and continue oxygen delivery.
10) As the bird awakes, take care to remove monitoring equipment and wrap the bird with a towel so that it can become sternal and stand. Extubation occurs when jaw tone returns and the bird's respirations return to a normal depth/frequency.

11) The bird should be returned to a heated, padded recovery cage (such as an incubator or critical care housing) and monitored until it is fully awake and ambulatory. A designated recovery nurse should stay with the bird for at least an hour to observe the bird.

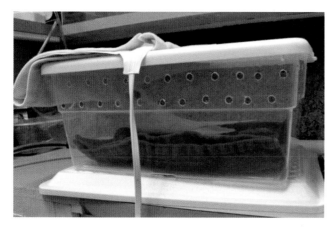

Figure 24.6 Heated recovery cage.

Rationale/Amplification

2, 4, 5: The avian anesthetist should have sufficient training and practice to be able to do this quickly, without injury to the glottis, and without forcing the beak open.

7: Staff on the surgery/anesthesia team must be trained in proper operation of the equipment and how to monitor for adverse readings.

11: The recovery period can be fairly rapid. One way to decrease injury to the bird recovering – they tend to flop around, flap their wings, but are ataxic and unbalanced and can injure themselves – wrap the bird loosely in a towel and place the bird in the darkened recovery cage. When it frees itself from the rolled towel, it is generally awake and no longer unbalanced. This is sometimes called "a birdie burrito," but works well. A designated recovery nurse must stay with the bird until it is fully awake and functioning normally. While in the hospital, it should be observed

Table 24.1 Commonly used analgesics in pet birds.

Agent	Dosage	Comments
Butorphanol	1–5 mg/kg IM, IV	Preemptive analgesia, often used in combination with midazolam for pre-anesthetic or analgesia/sedation for diagnostic procedures.
	2 mg/kg IN	Commonly used as part of analgesia/sedation in psittacines. Well-tolerated, no nasal irritation.
Fentanyl	0.2 mg/kg SC	Study in cockatoos, large dose and volume. Hyperactivity for first 15–30 min in some birds.
Gabapentin	3–10 mg/kg PO q 12–24 h	May initially have some sedation, titrate to effect for pain or feather destructive behavior decrease.
Meloxicam	1 mg/kg PO, IM, IV q 12–24 h	NSAID, PO lower bioavailability, provides analgesia by anti-inflammatory properties.
Tramadol	30 mg/kg PO q 6 h	Study in Hispaniolan Amazon parrots.

Source: References for Formulary Tables: Guzman DSM, Beaufrère H, Welle KR, Heatley J, Visser M, Harms CA. Birds. In: Carpenter JW, Harms CA (eds). Carpenter's Exotic Animal Formulary. Sixth Edition. 2023. Elsevier, St. Louis, MO. pp 222–443.

Table 24.2 Commonly used sedatives/pre-anesthetics in pet birds.

Agent	Dosage	Comments
Diazepam	2.5–4 mg/kg PO	Most species will cause some sedation. Used in combination with other drugs for pre-anesthesia. Can be reversed with flumazenil IN similarly to midazolam.
	5–30 mg/kg (ketamine) +0.5–2(D) mg/kg IV	Lower end of dosages preferred for sedation.
Midazolam	2 mg/kg IN	Parrots, higher doses needed in other species. Usually used in combination with butorphanol or ketamine. Can be reversed with flumazenil 0.05 mg/kg IN.
	2 mg/kg (M) plus 2 mg/kg butorphanol, IN	Adequate for many birds for diagnostic procedures or pre-anesthetic. This combination is often preferred and seems relatively safe even in ill birds.
	0.2–4 (M) mg/kg + 10–40 mg/kg (ketamine) SC, IM	Lower end of dosages preferred.
	1 (M) mg/kg + 10 (alfaxalone) mg/kg IM	May have longer recovery time than other combinations.

Source: References for Formulary Tables: Guzman DSM, Beaufrère H, Welle KR, Heatley J, Visser M, Harms CA. Birds. In: Carpenter JW, Harms CA (eds). Carpenter's Exotic Animal Formulary. Sixth Edition. 2023. Elsevier, St. Louis, MO. pp 222–443.

Table 24.3 Commonly used general anesthetics in pet birds.

Agent	Dosage	Comment
Isoflurane	3–5% induction; 1.5–2.5% maintenance	Titrate to depth needed. Usually administered with oxygen.
Propofol	5 mg/kg IV (induction), 1 mg/kg/min IV (maintenance)	IV sedative, hypnotic, used primarily for induction, but can be used IV for general anesthesia. Prolonged, variable recovery compared to isoflurane in the study on parrots.
Sevoflurane	5–6% induction, 1–4% maintenance	Similar to isoflurane for titrating for depth. Studies show slightly shorter recoveries with less ataxia. Administered with oxygen.

Source: References for Formulary Tables: Guzman DSM, Beaufrère H, Welle KR, Heatley J, Visser M, Harms CA. Birds. In: Carpenter JW, Harms CA (eds). Carpenter's Exotic Animal Formulary. Sixth Edition. 2023. Elsevier, St. Louis, MO. pp 222–443.

every 5–10 minutes for the next several hours. If the bird has had blood pressure, temperature, respiration/oxygenation, and heart rate stable and relatively similar to normal awake body parameters, anesthetic success is more likely.

BIBLIOGRAPHY

Guzman DSM, Beaufrère H, Welle KR, Heatley J, Visser M, Harms CA. Birds. In: Carpenter JW, Harms CA (eds). Carpenter's Exotic Animal Formulary. Sixth Edition. 2023. Elsevier, St. Louis, MO. pp 222–443.

Sabater Gonzalez M, Adams C. Psittacine sedation and anesthesia. 2022. *Vet Clin Exot Anim*; 25: 113–134.

Speer BL. Basic anaesthesia. In: Chitty J, Monks D (eds). *BSAVA Manual of Avian Practice. A Foundation Manual.* 2018. BSAVA, Quedgeley, UK. pp 232–241.

Appendix A

References and Resources

REFERENCE LIBRARY: RECOMMENDED AVIAN TEXTBOOKS

Chitty J, Monks D. (eds). *BSAVA Manual of Avian Practice: A Foundation Manual.* 2018. BSAVA, Quedgeley, UK.

Greenacre CB, Gerhardt L. Psittacines and passerine birds. In: Ballard B, Cheek R (eds). *Exotic Animal Medicine for the Veterinary Technician.* Third Edition. 2017. Wiley Blackwell, Ames, IA. pp 150–172.

Harrison GJ, Harrison LR. (eds). *Clinical Avian Medicine and Surgery. Including Aviculture.* 1986. WB Saunders Company, Philadelphia, PA.

Harrison GJ, Lightfoot TL. (eds). *Clinical Avian Medicine, Volumes I, II.* 2006. Spix Publishing, Palm Beach, FL.

King AS, McLelland J. *Birds: Their Structure and Function.* 1984. Balliere Tindall, Philadelphia, PA.

Phalen DN, Baron H. Passerines. In: Graham JE, Doss GA, Beaufrere J (eds). Exotic Animal Emergency and Critical Care Medicine. 2021 Wiley Blackwell, Ames, IA. pp 1551–1569 (ebook paging).

Ritchie BW, Harrison GJ, Harrison LR. Avian Medicine: Principles and Application. 1994. Wingers Publishing, Lake Worth, FL.

Sirois M. Birds. Laboratory Animal and Exotic Pet Medicine. Principles and Procedures. Second Edition. 2016. *Elsevier*, St. Louis, MO. pp 35–67.

Speer BL (ed). Current Therapy in Avian Medicine and Surgery. First Edition. 2016. Elsevier, St. Louis, MO.

Wyre NR. Psittacines. In: Graham JE, Doss GA, Beaufrere J (eds). Exotic Animal Emergency and Critical Care Medicine. 2021. Wiley Blackwell, Ames, IA. pp 1491–1550 (ebook paging).

JOURNALS

Journal of Avian Medicine and Surgery

https://www.aav.org/page/jams Member benefit
https://bioone.org/journals/journal-of-avian-medicine-and-surgery

Journal of Exotic Pet Medicine

https://aemv.org/ Member benefit
https://www.sciencedirect.com/journal/journal-of-exotic-pet-medicine
https://www.us.elsevierhealth.com/journal-of-exotic-pet-medicine-1557-5063.html

Veterinary Clinics North America: Exotic Animal Practice

https://www.vetexotic.theclinics.com/
https://www.sciencedirect.com/journal/veterinary-clinics-of-north-america-exotic-animal-practice

On-Line Networking

- Exotic DVM Forum: free, open to veterinarians and veterinary students. www.exoticdvm.com.
- Veterinary Information Network: requires paid membership to access avian, exotic discussion groups and CE. https://www.vin.com/vin/default.aspx?pid=130&meta=108&id=0
- Association of Avian Veterinarians has many online educational opportunities. Membership required. www.aav.org.

Appendix B

Abbreviations

AO	aortic outflow
BP	blood pressure
BPM	breaths per minute or beats per minute
CPR	cardiopulmonary resuscitation
CT	computed tomography
D3	vitamin D 3
Diast	diastole
DV	dorso-ventral
E collar	Elizabethan collar
ECG	electrocardiograph
ET	endotracheal tube
Exam	examination
FNA	fine needle aspirate
g	gram
Ga	gauge
IC	intracoelomic
IM	intramuscular
IN	intranasal
IO	intraosseous
IPPV	intermittent positive pressure ventilation
IU	international units
IV	intravenous
kg	kilogram
L	left
LA	left atrium
Lat	lateral
LV	left ventricle
mg	milligram
mL	milliliter
MRI	magnetic resonance imaging
NSAID	nonsteroidal anti-inflammatory drug
PCR	polymerase chain reaction
PO	per os
q (a number) h	every (a number) of hours (Latin: Quaque horas)

Manual of Clinical Procedures in Pet Birds, First Edition. Cathy A. Johnson-Delaney and Tracy Bennett.
© 2025 John Wiley & Sons, Inc. Published 2025 by John Wiley & Sons, Inc.
Companion website: www.wiley.com/go/johnson-delaney/manual

R	right
RA	right atrium
RV	right ventricle
SC	subcutaneous
Sys	systole
UVB	ultraviolet B light
VD	ventro-dorsal

Appendix C

Common Pet and Aviary Birds

This list is only some of the many species that may be seen in pet and aviary practice. Scientific names can change with time as genetic investigations continue. Many species have multiple names in the pet trade, so it is advantageous to record the scientific name in the patient's record.

Common Name	Scientific Name
Passerifomes	
Blue-capped cordon-bleu (finch)	*Uraeginthus cyanocephalus*
Canary, domestic	*Serinus canaria domestica*
Gouldian finch (Lady Gouldian)	*Erythrura gouldiae*
Java Rice Bird (Java sparrow)	*Padda oryzivora*
Mynah (Hill)	*Gracula religiosa*
Society finch (Bengalese, Bengali finch)	*Lonchura striata domestica*
Zebra finch	*Taeniopygia guttata*
Psittaciformes	
Amazon parrots	
Blue-fronted Amazon	*Amazona aestiva*
Double Yellow-headed Amazon	*Amazona oratix* ssp
Mealy Amazon	*Amazona farinosa*
Orange-winged Amazon	*Amazona amazonica*
Hispaniolan Amazon	*Amazona ventralis*
Mexican red-crowned Amazon	*Amazona viridigenalis*
Yellow-fronted Amazon (Yellow-crowned)	*Amazona ochrocephalia*
Yellow-naped Amazon	*Amazona (oratrix) auropalliata*
Cockatoos	
Galah (Rose-breasted)	*Eolophus roseicapilla*
Goffin's cockatoo	*Cacatua goffini*
Greater sulphur-crested cockatoo	*Cacatua galerita galerita*
Lesser sulphur-crested cockatoo	*Cacatua sulphurea*
Bare-eyed cockatoo (Little Corella)	*Cacatua sanguinea*

(Continued)

Manual of Clinical Procedures in Pet Birds, First Edition. Cathy A. Johnson-Delaney and Tracy Bennett.
© 2025 John Wiley & Sons, Inc. Published 2025 by John Wiley & Sons, Inc.
Companion website: www.wiley.com/go/johnson-delaney/manual

Common Name	Scientific Name
Major Mitchell's cockatoo (Pink, Leadbeater's)	*Lophochroa leadbeateri*
Moluccan cockatoo	*Cacatua moluccensis*
Sulphur-crested cockatoo	*Cacatua galerita*
Umbrella cockatoo (White)	*Cacatua alba*
Conures	
Blue-crowned	*Thectocercus acuticaudatus*
Green-cheeked	*Pyrrhura molinae*
Jenday (Jendaya)	*Aratinga jandaya*
Mitred	*Psittacara mitratus*
Nanday	*Nandayus nenday*
Patagonian	*Cyanoliseus patagonus*
Sun	*Aratinga solstitialis*
Small parrots	
Budgerigar (Parakeet, budgie)	*Melopsittacus undulatus*
Cockatiel	*Nymphicus hollandicus*
Black-masked lovebird	*Agapornis personatus*
Fischer's lovebird	*Agapornis fischeri*
Peach-faced lovebird	*Agapornis roseicollis*
Lories and lorikeets	
Black-capped lory	*Lorius lory*
Rainbow lorikeet	*Trichoglossus moluccanus*
Red lory	*Eos bornea borneo (formerly E. rosea)*
Macaws	
Blue and gold	*Ara ararauna*
Catalina (Rainbow)	*Ara ararauna X Ara macao*
Green-winged	*Ara chloroptera*
Harlequin	*Ara ararauna X Ara chloroptera*
Hyacinth	*Anodorhynchus hyacinthus*
Military	*Ara militaris*
Scarlet	*Ara macao*
Yellow-naped (Yellow-collared)	*Primolius auricollis*
Other common psittacines	
African grey parrot	*Psittacus erithacus*
Timneh African grey parrot	*Psittacus erithacus timneh*
Black-headed (Black-capped) caique	*Pionites melanocephalus*
Blue-headed pionus	*Pionus menstruus*
Eastern rosella	*Platycercus eximius*
Eclectus parrot	*Eclectus roratus*
Hawk-headed parrot	*Deroptyus accipitrinus*

Common Name	Scientific Name
Indian ring-necked parakeet	*Psittacula krameri*
Maximilian pionus	*Pionus maximiliani*
Meyer's parrot	*Poicephalus meyeri*
Monk (Quaker) parakeet	*Myiopsitta monachus*
Senegal parrot	*Poicephalus rufiventris*
White-capped pionus	*Pionus senilis*

Index

Manual of Clinical Procedures in Pet Birds, First Edition. Cathy A. Johnson-Delaney and Tracy Bennett.
© 2025 John Wiley & Sons, Inc. Published 2025 by John Wiley & Sons, Inc.
Companion website: www.wiley.com/go/johnson-delaney/manual